Getting into

Dental School

Getting Into guides

Getting into

Dental
School

Adam Cross

7th edition

trotman | **t**

Getting into Dental School

This 7th edition published in 2011 by Trotman Publishing, an imprint of Crimson Publishing Limited, Westminster House, Kew Road, Richmond, Surrey TW9 2ND

© Trotman Publishing 2011

Author: Adam Cross

6th edn by Steven Piumatti published in 2009
5th edn by James Burnett published in 2007
4th edn by James Burnett & Andrew Long published in 2005
3rd edn by James Burnett & Andrew Long published in 2003
2nd edn by Joe Ruston & James Burnett in 2000
1st edn by Joe Ruston in 1996

Editions 1–6 published by Trotman and Co Ltd

British Library Cataloguing in Publication Data
A catalogue record for this book is available from the British Library.

ISBN 978 1 84455 389 1

Typeset by IDSUK (Data Connection) Ltd.
Printed and bound in the UK by Ashford Colour Press, Gosport, Hants.

Contents

Contents

About the author

Adam Cross is Assistant Principal at independent college MPW Birmingham and has several years' expertise in helping students gain entry onto competitive undergraduate courses such as dentistry and medicine. In addition to his careers guidance expertise, Adam also helps students with pre-admissions tests such as the UK Clinical Aptitude Test (UKCAT). Adam is a highly regarded teacher of biology and his commitment to pedagogy ensures that he keeps up to date with developments in the fields of science and teaching and learning.

Acknowledgements

I would firstly like to thank Mark Shingleton for his guidance and support over recent months, as well as his contributions to the content of the book. I would also like to thank Neelam Hussain, Joy Harrild, Sameera Mukadam, Andrew Jones, Samera Altaf, Joanne Lamb and Jo White, as well as numerous others, for giving me an insight into life as a dental student, and Dr George Mitchell, Dr Tom Fraser and Dr Neva Patel for giving me an insight into the world of dentistry. In addition, I would like to thank the admissions teams from all of the UK dental schools who put up with my countless emails and phone calls, as well as the British Dental Association and the British Dental Health Foundation for providing factual material relating to dental careers. Finally, I would like to thank both my wife and daughter for their support while I was writing the book

I would like to emphasise here that although the information in the book has been provided by experts, most of the views expressed are my own, and any mistakes are also mine.

Adam Cross
February 2011

Introduction

If you have picked up this book, it probably means that you are considering applying to study dentistry and so ultimately want to become a dentist. At this stage of the process, you may be unsure about the details of how to apply, or how best to prepare yourself for an admissions interview. You may have no idea about the type of work experience you will be required to have or the demands of pre-admissions tests. However, the whole purpose of this book is to guide you through the process step by step and ensure that you are prepared to make a successful application and secure your place at university.

This book is divided into the following chapters, which will guide you through each stage of the process.

Chapter 1 focuses on the research you need to do before applying. This is divided between research into universities and potential courses and research into dentistry as a career.

Chapter 2 describes the structure of undergraduate courses and the options for study beyond this. It also gives information on possible sources of funding for undergraduate students.

Chapter 3 deals with preparing your application to make it as attractive as possible to admissions tutors. It includes advice on how to choose a dental school and the UCAS application procedure, including how to write an effective personal statement. It also deals with the UK Clinical Aptitude Test (UKCAT) and how best to prepare for it.

Chapter 4 provides advice on how to prepare for interview and impress the admissions tutors. It also gives some examples of the types of questions that you may be asked.

Chapter 5 looks at the options you have on results day and describes the steps that you need to take if you miss the grades or do not hold any offers.

Chapter 6 gives information about international students applying to study dentistry, but also deals with applications from other non-standard applicants, such as mature students, graduates, students who have studied arts A levels, and retake students.

Chapter 7 looks at career options in dentistry and the different pathways that a dentist could follow. It also looks at your graduate prospects as a dentist and what typical earnings are.

Chapter 8 provides key information on some current dental issues, such as mouth cancer, fluoridation of water and NHS dentistry.

Finally, in Chapter 9, there are tables providing further information and statistics on dentistry admissions.

There are a number of case studies provided throughout the book to support the material being discussed. This information is designed to illustrate the appropriate points and should give you an opportunity to see the issues under consideration demonstrated. Like other books in this series, such as *Getting into Medical School*, this title is designed to be a route map for potential dentists rather than a guide to dentistry as a profession. Further information on issues related to being a dentist can be found on websites such as the British Dental Association's (the BDA – see www.bda.org), or directly from your own dentist.

Entrance requirements have been given primarily in terms of A level grades throughout the book; information for students who have studied Scottish Highers, the International Baccalaureate (IB) and other qualifications is given in Chapter 3.

What role do dentists have in society?

As you have probably already realised, dentistry involves much more than gazing into people's mouths all day! It is a challenging vocation which requires a wide range of skills to be mastered if you are going to be successful.

So why do people choose to study dentistry? Dental professionals often cite a number of reasons for pursuing dentistry as a career. These include:

- developing their interest in human biology and dental issues
- helping and improving people's well-being and confidence, from the very young to the aged
- being a positive and helpful part of the community
- working with your hands, and being able to demonstrate high levels of manual skill
- working with a wide range of people on a day-to-day basis
- freedom to choose your own patients
- an opportunity to run a business and be your own boss
- flexibility in choosing the length of the working day
- working as part of a team
- status and respect
- money.

Dentistry is definitely not just about teeth, but also about oral health in general. Dentists are increasingly filling a much wider societal role than they once had historically; in addition to carrying out standard treatments, as oral professionals and health practitioners they look after the well-being of their patients and thus become an important part of any community. Take, for example, the advice that a dentist has to give to patients in relation to good oral health. This may include information and advice on diet, giving up smoking and its possible knock-on effects for general health, and recommendations about courses of treatment.

The British Dental Health Foundation, which is associated with the International Health Foundation, has an interesting website that outlines the variety of issues that dentists have to deal with when treating patients on a daily basis. These include obvious issues such as dental decay and sensitive teeth, but also more wide-ranging themes such as mouth cancer, diet and bad breath (www.dentalhealth.org.uk/faqs/browseleaflets.php). A quick look through this site should give you an insight into the range of skills that a modern dentist needs.

Take for example the skills required to deal with patients with special needs. Those with physical disabilities may need assistance to get into the dental chair, while people with learning disabilities may become distressed at the thought of going to the dentist and require extra time to be reassured and appropriately cared for. Some patients may have other special needs, such as communication difficulties or being visually or hearing impaired. People with severe medical problems may also need extra care in order to be treated safely and successfully. A dentist must take account of all these and have the skills to deal with them when providing dental care. A dentist may even have to make different arrangements to meet the needs of the individual, and often home visits will need to be organised. The salaried primary care dental service (SPCDS) in the UK today is responsible for the treatment of people with special medical or social needs, such as complex medical problems, disabilities or mental health problems, who are unable to be treated by general dental practitioners (GDPs). In these cases, some dentists (or community dental officers) are willing to work in a more peripatetic fashion than a full-time surgery environment, and the patient's dentist is responsible for referring them to the local clinic, with any hospital letters and X-rays, to give the community dental officer an idea of the patient's dental history.

Another major aspect of the role that dentists have in society is education. Along with dental nurses they are at the forefront of teaching the public about good dental hygiene. There is a major push for preventive dentistry by the NHS and dentists today. The focus is to promote long-term care of the mouth, teeth, gums and cheeks, and extends, as mentioned earlier, to advice on areas such as diet. Teaching awareness of oral health and hygiene is of paramount importance. Dentists educate patients on caring for teeth and gums by encouraging them to use fluorides, flossing and brushing. Teaching through direct consultations or by the pamphlets available in surgeries are just some of the ways that this can be achieved, with others including the education of young people in schools, and educating elderly people in nursing homes about keeping dentures clean and viable. This is all carried out by dentists and oral health advisors working in the SPCDS.

Ultimately, the goal of educating the population about oral health and preventive dentistry is to keep the need for major dental treatment to a minimum by maintaining a healthy mouth. As the two major causes of tooth loss are tooth decay and gum disease, the better people prevent or deal with these two problems the more chance they have of keeping their teeth for life. The joint efforts of the dentist, the hygienist and the patient can help to prevent the need for treatment, and so avoid the traditional pattern of fillings and extractions. This is a saving not only to the individual in terms of time and money but also to the community in the long term.

Dentists are often the first to spot medical problems that might otherwise go unnoticed until the problem has worsened. One example of this is oral cancer. There are more than 5,000 new cases of oral cancer each year, and about 1,800 of these patients die from the disease (http://info.cancerresearchuk.org/cancerstats/types/oral/?a=5441). The role of the dentist is vital in the early diagnosis of the disease and referral for appropriate treatment. Dentists are also the first people to recognise other problems such as ulcers and cold sores that could lead to more serious conditions. As with all disease, early recognition is more than half the battle.

Over recent years, the field of cosmetic dentistry has also been an area of rapid growth, with dentists playing an increasing role in providing cosmetic improvement for the public. This was an area of growth strongly commented on by the dentists with whom I spoke while researching this book. Not only is it increasing their scope but it is also a lucrative area in our image-conscious society. Cosmetic dental surgery involves treatments to straighten, lighten, reshape and repair teeth. This can also include veneers, crowns, bridges, tooth-coloured fillings, implants and tooth whitening and correction of bites. For example, as people get older, a face can sag, the chin can stick out and the smile droop if the 'bite' is not corrected – what dentists refer to as 'face collapse'. It can even cause headaches, neck pain and other pains in the body. Thus, there is a need for rectification. Usually, obvious abnormal 'bites' or crooked teeth are fixed early in childhood, but today even mild forms of the above are now seen as a problem and more young and mature adults than before are undergoing this type of cosmetic treatment.

What are the necessary attributes of a dentist?

As with any competitive university course and vocation, candidates must be able to demonstrate not only academic ability and the right personal qualities but also commitment if they wish to succeed. Practising dentists, admissions tutors and current students all agree that demonstrating dedication to dentistry is of paramount importance during the application process, during university study and beyond into a dentist's professional life.

It is therefore vital that an applicant to a dentistry course is certain that they want to become a dentist before applying. Wanting to study dentistry because 'you like science' or because 'you want to earn lots of money' is unlikely to be enough to convince an admissions tutor to give you a place. It is also unlikely to be enough to keep you motivated throughout your career.

Dentistry, unlike medicine, offers fewer diverse pathways or opportunities later on in your career. This ultimately means that you must be fully informed about what the career path entails because it is difficult to move effortlessly into something else without some degree of re-specialisation.

In addition to being fully committed to dentistry, a dentist must also be able to demonstrate the following:

- the ability to successfully communicate with patients
- an enjoyment of dealing with people and working in a team
- an ability to reassure patients who are scared or in pain
- a caring and sympathetic nature and immense patience
- a high degree of manual dexterity
- self-motivation
- an enjoyment of science and developments in the field of dentistry
- an excellent memory and an ability to solve problems
- versatility
- mental and physical stamina – remember, a dentist may have to concentrate on a single task for hours
- the ability to multi-task – this is necessary for running a business
- an ability to train and manage people and get the best out of them.

Some of the above qualities will not surprise you. It would be hard to be a successful dentist if you could not bear to be around other people, and unsympathetic dentists end up with few patients. Similarly, if you do not enjoy science, you would be unlikely to gain the necessary grades at A level or pass your exams at university. But often overlooked is the need for manual dexterity; dentistry is probably not a course for you to pursue if you are a particularly clumsy person!

If you believe that you have the above qualities, the next step is to investigate what being a dentist is actually like and to find out what they do. In brief, a dentist's job includes tasks such as filling cavities, examining X-rays, applying protective sealant on teeth, extracting teeth, removing decay, and taking measurements and making models for dentures. They also often treat gum disease by performing surgery on patients. As you can see, this is where versatility is needed – and stamina. Patience and empathy are also much-needed attributes, as every day a dentist will be working with their patients and their staff.

Many people are unaware that dentists are usually self-employed, and the amount of money they earn is directly related to the number of patients they see. Without stamina and self-motivation, you are unlikely, at least at the start of your career, to earn as much as you might hope.

A recent survey revealed that the average student debt on graduating was almost £30,000. Many of the students surveyed had multiple debts, including student loans, bank loans, overdrafts, credit cards and debts to parents; the most common types of debt were student and bank loans. Therefore, once qualified, dentists, not surprisingly, need to earn enough not only to support themselves but also to begin paying off their debts.

Are there any downsides to being a dentist?

There are, of course, some negative aspects of dentistry. In its highly informative advice sheet on careers in dentistry, the BDA urges prospective dentists to consider a number of factors including stress, lack of job and financial security (because of self-employment), lack of career progression, aggressive or frightened patients and last, but by no means least, the boredom that can accompany repetitive routine tasks. If you are worried about any of these, you should talk to your own dentist to see how he or she feels about them. Some dentists will warn students against going into the profession without being aware that dentistry suits people who are prepared to work hard and who enjoy being with other people.

Before looking at the applications and admissions processes in more detail, you may be interested to read what a dental student who has recently begun her course had to say about her choice of career thus far. Bear in mind that this could be you in one or two years' time.

Case study 1: Neelam Hussain

Neelam Hussain is currently a second-year student at Birmingham University.

'Throughout my education I considered pursuing a number of different careers, including dermatology, hairdressing and even TV presenting! I started considering dentistry after I had attended a careers convention at my secondary school. I then spent time researching the details of dentistry as a course and a career and realised how interesting the subject was.

'Following this, I proceeded to organise work experience so that I could get a first-hand feel for what it was like to be a dentist. I found it very difficult to arrange a placement at first, as I had no contacts in my family or among my friends, but after contacting numerous dental practices, I was able to secure two placements. My first was a two-week placement at a general dental practice and my second was a three-day placement at a community dental practice.

'I learnt a great deal from my work experience and this really did confirm for me that I wanted to apply to study dentistry. During my work experience at the GDP, I was able to have hands-on experience in developing X-rays and preparing to take impressions for dentures and crowns. Working in a community dental practice demonstrated the vast differences that exist between different types of practice. In particular, I was able to see how dealing with patients suffering from other illnesses affected the approach the dentist took. It also allowed me to see that putting the patient at ease is essential to good-quality dental care.'

Neelam decided to study A level Biology, Chemistry and Mathematics and AS Art and Design and achieved AAAB grades. Following her results, she took up her place at Birmingham University.

'My experience of the course so far has been very exciting. It is very different to school and studying for A levels as there is a lot more work involved. However, the work we undertake is very interesting, which means I don't always see it as work but enjoy doing it! My first year was mainly biology-based, which was great for me as I like biology. However, there was not a massive emphasis on specific dental theory. I did appreciate the small bits of dental work we did such as composite fillings on models of teeth as well as observation sessions at the dental school. So far, it has been fascinating to learn about the anatomy of the body, as well as different bodily systems, which I didn't think I would learn about in dental school. It is not all concentrated on the facial area; it goes much further! In addition to this, the people on the course really do make it appealing and bring out the fun element of the subject.

'To anybody thinking about studying dentistry, I would say definitely do it! The experience I have had so far has been wonderful. Make sure that you do lots of interview preparation, research hot topics related to dentistry and make sure you demonstrate the knowledge you have in your interview.'

1 | What do I need to do before applying?

According to UCAS, in 2009 there were 3,720 applicants for entry into dentistry competing for 1,215 places, a ratio of 2.72 applicants per place. Of this, the ratio of women to men was about 56:44, and the number of places gained by women was slightly higher than those gained by men, with a success rate of 39% (714 accepts from 1,854 applications) in comparison with 35% (501 acceptances from 1,450 applications), respectively. In other words, women were, on average, slightly more successful than men in their applications. This might be due to a more mature approach, better preparation and focus and better AS level grades, or it may just be due to chance.

Around 459 of the total number of applicants were from overseas, and only 65 were accepted. It is more difficult to get a successful application through if you are an overseas applicant, and the reasons for this are discussed further in Chapter 6.

The 2009 numbers signal an increase in the number of applications on previous years, so the forecast, based on current trends, is for applica-tion numbers to continue rising – thus increasing the competition for places. This will make AS grades and thorough preparation even more important in coming years, as there will be more competition for the limited number of available places. Table 3 in Chapter 9 (see page 111) gives an indication of the 2009 and most recent 2010 application num-bers; however, it does not give the number of places available in 2010 as this information was not available at the time of writing.

It is worth mentioning here that in the round of applications for 2010 entry there was an increase in total applicants from 3,304 to 3,720, a rise of 12.6% compared with the 2009 applications (including EU and non-EU applicants). It is also worth noting that between 2006 and 2010 there has been a 27.8% increase in total applications for dentistry courses, with the greatest increase coming from female applicants (see Table 5, Chapter 9, page 113). This expansion in application numbers is consistent with the general rise in higher education applications over recent years and further demonstrates the need for thorough prepara-tion when applying for dentistry.

Lastly, in 2009 there were a significant number of students who narrowly missed their offers and therefore the opportunity to take up their place.

Under similar circumstances for other courses, such as biological sciences, the place would be offered to other prospective students via the UCAS Clearing system after results day in mid-August. However, when considering a competitive course such as dentistry, it is virtually unheard of that there would be any places on offer in Clearing. This means that getting a place on a dentistry course through Clearing should not be considered a viable route. This is because the number of offers given in the first place is often greater than the actual number of places available. For example, the University of Glasgow made 148 offers for Dentistry in 2009 but finally accepted only 92 students. This situation is mirrored by all universities and aims to ensure that the course is filled once students who do not get the required grades or who decide to go to another university have been discounted.

Exploring the options

So what are the steps that you need to take to ensure that you have an excellent chance of being selected for an interview and offered a place?

The first step is to thoroughly research the stages of the application process and the demands of the course and career. This is vital for a number of reasons. You need:

- to see whether dentistry is the right career for you
- to see whether your personal and academic skills are matched to the course
- to find out which universities offer dentistry and to which you want to apply
- to find out the details of courses offered by each university and the one that might best suit you (while the courses may have the same title, their structures can be vastly different)
- to give you ideas and information about possible work experience placements
- to find out what makes an excellent personal statement
- to understand the demands of the interview process and to help develop interview skills.

Ideally, your research should start in your AS year or even earlier. Most schools start a programme of UCAS and career prospects-related workshops halfway through the AS year, with the aim being that students should have a clear idea where they want to apply to after the summer holidays. However, you should make your mind up about study-ing dentistry as soon as possible to give you the maximum amount of time for research and work experience placements.

There are several areas that need to be considered in your research. These can be divided into:

- media research – internet, books, periodicals and specialist magazines
- discussion with professionals
- work experience.

Some suggestions for media research are given below.

Internet

- The UCAS website (www.ucas.ac.uk) is very useful for research into degree courses and gives lots of details about the entry requirements and course structure at each university.
- Newspaper sites – the *Guardian* (www.guardian.co.uk/education) and *The Times* (www.thetimes.co.uk) provide useful information about university league tables and subject rankings.
- www.mpw.co.uk/getintomed – this website provides links to sites such as the Department of Health and World Health Organization.
- The British Dental Association (www.bda.org) gives information primarily on topical issues for healthcare professionals.
- The British Dental Health Foundation (www.dentalhealth.org) focuses more on raising public awareness of important oral hygiene issues. Both websites are useful if you want to gain a wider understanding of current issues.
- www.dentistry.co.uk – this is an online periodical that is very useful for up-to-date information about the field of dentistry.
- University websites – most of the information you will need about applying to a university and about the course can be found on individual universities' websites. These are a treasure trove of information and will help you get a feel for each institution and the nature of the course it is offering.

Books and periodicals

- *HEAP 2012: University Degree Course Offers* by Brian Heap has a short section on dentistry and the universities offering dentistry courses, and gives a good overview of entry requirements.
- University prospectuses – calling universities and asking them to send you their prospectus will help you get a feel for the institution and the course. Note that a number of universities have full prospectuses online.
- Subscribing to magazines such as *The Dentist* will let you find out first-hand about issues and developments in dentistry. This would be seen as extracurricular reading and would demonstrate your interest to university admissions panels.

Work experience

Discussing your interest in dentistry with dentists working in the field is an excellent way of gathering first-hand information about the subject. It may be a good idea to start by talking to your own local dentist or any family members or friends that are dentists. Ask them as many questions as you can think of about studying dentistry at university and about the career options for dentists. Make sure you ask about the positives and negatives of the job, as practising dentists are the individuals who are best placed to answer these questions honestly. It would also be worth asking about any interesting current issues in dentistry.

However, by far the best thing you can do to decide whether dentistry is for you is to organise, either by yourself and/or via your school, some work experience in a practice, where you will be able to work-shadow a dentist. This should answer any questions you may have and will also give you an opportunity to find out what goes on in a dental surgery and some of the responsibilities that a dentist has to fulfil. Remember, gaining relevant work experience is not just a desirable part of your application, it is a prerequisite for most courses; it is unlikely that you will be considered unless you have evidence of this. Even more importantly, work experience is a chance for you to decide whether dentistry is the right career for you. I have seen a number of students who have expressed a desire to be a dentist but then totally changed their mind after a week of shadowing and observation. Conversely, I have also seen many students who have shown increased dedication in pursuing dentistry following work experience.

Most admissions tutors agree that the absolute minimum amount of time that prospective dental students should spend work-shadowing dentists is two weeks; anything less than this and you will be unlikely to appreciate the realities of dentistry as a career. However, as the admissions process becomes increasingly competitive, most admissions tutors want you to demonstrate an ongoing commitment to the field of dentistry. This means that you should ideally aim to spend time with several different dentists on a regular basis over a number of months. Simply carrying out the basic two weeks is unlikely to display the required commitment. This fact alone means that preparation for your application to study dentistry needs to start as soon as possible, preferably in your AS year or earlier; if you only decide on dentistry as a career at the start of your A2 year, it will leave little or no time to build up a solid portfolio of work experience. In addition to undertaking work experience directly related to dentistry, it is also desirable to show evidence of experience or voluntary work in a care-based environment; for example, a hospital, a children's hospice or a nursing home. This will also help to develop your understanding of the wider world and other clinical environments and strengthen your application.

How to arrange work experience

If you are lucky, your school will have a scheme whereby it can organise some work experience for you. The disadvantage is that you will then be unable to impress the selectors with your dynamism and determination as you will not be able to say that you arranged the work experience yourself. However, even where work experience schemes exist, it is unlikely that they will provide every placement for you, and so at some point you will have to demonstrate initiative in making the necessary arrangements. There are two routes that you should try: approaching local dentists, or making use of contacts that your friends or family may have.

In order to approach local dentists about possible work experience, you should first get the names and addresses of local dental practices from a website such as the Yellow Pages (www.yell.co.uk) or the BDA (www.bda.org). You should then write a formal letter, and include the name of a referee; that is, someone who can vouch for your interest in dentistry as well as your reliability. Your careers teacher, housemaster/housemistress or form teacher would be ideal. An example of a suitable letter is given in the box below.

52 Boscombe Road
Shufflefield
SH3 2DS

Mr M. Littlewood [You should telephone the practice for the name of one of the dentists.]
Sparkling Smile Dental Clinic
17 Poole Crescent
Shufflefield
SH15 3AB

1 October 2010

Dear Mr Littlewood

I am currently in my first year of studying A levels in Biology, Chemistry, Maths and Psychology at Shufflefield School, and I am interested in pursuing a career in dentistry. I was wondering if it would be possible to meet you to discuss what the profession is like and then perhaps spend a week shadowing you or one of your colleagues, so that I can get some first-hand experience?

If you require a reference, please contact my form tutor, Mr Jones. His contact details are as follows:

Mr T Jones
Shufflefield School
Shufflefield
SH21 2CF

I look forward to hearing from you.

Yours sincerely

Mr Robert Smith

Shadowing dentists is useful for a number of reasons:

- it will help you to decide whether you really want to be a dentist
- it will demonstrate your commitment to studying dentistry to admissions tutors
- you may, if you can demonstrate to the dentist that you are serious about dentistry, be able to ask him or her for a reference in the future.

Things to look out for during work experience

Your work experience will provide you with invaluable opportunities to develop your knowledge and understanding of dentistry as a career. It is therefore vital that you pay close attention to what is going on around you so you can get the most from the experience. It is a good idea to carry a notebook and pen so that you can jot down answers to questions you have asked as well as any thoughts or observations related to your experiences. In addition, it is worth trying to keep a diary of what you have observed as this will be an invaluable resource when it comes to writing a personal statement and attending interviews.

Make sure you are as professional as possible throughout your placements; dress as the dentists dress, be clean, tidy and reasonably formal. Ask intelligent questions to further your understanding of what is going on. Offer to help the dentist or the receptionists with routine tasks. Show an interest in all that is going on around you, bearing in mind that this might be your job in a few years' time.

During your placements, pay attention to the following aspects of dental practice.

The attributes of a dentist

Dentists need to be much more than dental treatment robots; it is therefore a good idea to keep a note of the range of characteristics the dentist demonstrates on a day-to-day basis as well as the variety of tasks they carry out. This will help provide you with a list of the sort of skills you will need to develop as a dentist and will ultimately help you in developing the knowledge of dentists required for a successful interview.

Interactions with patients

A vital part of the dentist's role is to interact with patients to discuss potential treatment routes and to guide and reassure them. Take time to observe how a dentist communicates with patients, particularly those who are anxious about being treated.

The variety of treatments available to patients

Make sure that you know what you are observing during your placement. Ask the dentist or nurse for the technical names of the procedures you see, and for information on the materials and equipment used. Ask about the advantages and disadvantages of different types of filling, implant or denture.

Make sure that you are aware not only of the way that damaged teeth are repaired, but also about preventive dentistry, orthodontics and oral hygiene. You should also try to discuss the dentist's role in identifying other problems, such as mouth cancer.

The roles of different team members

In any dental setting, there will be a wide range of individuals involved who are vital to the overall functioning of the team. For example, in addition to the dentist there may also be dental nurses, hygienists, receptionists and administrators. Make sure you take time to talk to as many members of the team as possible and ask them about the role they play.

Working as a dentist

Ask the dentist about his or her life. Find out about the hours, the way in which dentists are paid, the demands of the job and the career options. Find out what dentists like about the job and what they dislike.

Ultimately, being observant and asking questions will help you further your understanding of what is required in being a dentist. At the end of each of your placements, you should ask yourself whether this is still a career path that you wish to pursue. If there are any aspects of the work that you dislike, ask yourself whether these would put you off becoming a dentist.

Case study 2: Joy Harrild

Joy is currently in her second year at Birmingham University. After careful research into her career options, Joy felt that dentistry was the only one that really stood out. She was excited about the fact that the course was based on developing communication and practical skills as well as learning scientific theory, and was particularly interested in the patient-centred nature of the profession. In preparation for her application, Joy work-shadowed an orthodontist, took placements at a private and an NHS general practice and attended a dental biomaterials course at Queen Mary University. Together, these helped her understand the demands of the profession and fostered her desire to pursue this career path.

'My range of work experience taught me loads of things about dentistry and how it works: the importance of communication skills, time management and professionalism. It also gave me an insight into new developments in the NHS and some tips for applying to dentistry courses.'

Joy went on to achieve AAA grades in Biology, Chemistry and English Literature at A level and as a result was able to take up her place at Birmingham University.

'The dentistry course at Birmingham is undeniably hard work, but when you reach the stage where you start practical work and apply all the knowledge you've gained over the course, everything starts to click together. The satisfaction from that feeling is great and is only going to get better when you have your own patients.'

Joy's particular areas of interest at this point lie in dealing with people. 'At the moment, I particularly enjoy the behavioural science and communication skills as these are directly related to dealing with patients.' Ultimately, she would like to develop her interest in working with and treating mentally ill and disabled patients.

Joy's advice to aspiring dentists: 'Work hard, be enthusiastic and don't give up!'

2 | What is it like to study dentistry?

Undergraduate

Studying dentistry in the UK should be a challenging but highly rewarding experience, as the provision at British dental schools is normally first rate. Prospective students should be aware from the outset that attending dental school will require commitment and dedication; ask any current dental student and they will tell you how much hard work is needed to succeed. Undergraduate dental courses last for five years and at the end of their studies students will gain the initials BDS or BChD (the Latin equivalent of BDS) after their name. There is no distinction between these two classifications as both refer to a Bachelor of Dental Surgery; the distinction depends on the dental school that a student has attended.

Most of the dental schools adopt a similar structure in their courses but key differences have begun to emerge in the teaching methodology and delivery of course content. It is therefore important for students to carefully research the details of each course and appreciate the key features. This is obviously vital in selecting an appropriate dental school, submitting a relevant personal statement and preparing for an interview. Many of the dental schools have begun to put a greater emphasis on students taking responsibility for their own learning. At Leeds, for example, much emphasis is placed on students undertaking self-directed learning.

Universities teach in a range of ways, from traditional large lectures to small tuition groups of around eight. A number of schools, such as Liverpool and Manchester, have successfully developed courses that have elements of problem-based learning (PBL) at their core. Many of the dental schools have begun to place a greater responsibility on students to be accountable for their own learning, and prospective students should be aware of terms such as self-directed learning. These approaches are designed to develop an independent and inquisitive approach to learning, using libraries and discussing issues with colleagues to solve problems (as the name suggests). Bristol, by contrast, does not subscribe to the PBL approach, and adopts what it calls a traditional integrated programme of lectures and seminars supported by opportunities to learn in a more clinical setting. Some courses integrate elements of clinical contact from the first year of the course, while others do not introduce clinical contact until year two or three. At Cardiff, for example, first-year students will have exposure to clinical contact for half a day per week, whereas at Birmingham clinical teaching and patient treatment begins at the end of the second year. As you would expect, all dental schools are committed to using up-to-date technology to help teach the curriculum, and students will notice how keen the various dental schools are to demonstrate this during open days.

The reason why a dental course lasts five years is that the teaching covers a wide variety of elements. Most dental schools will normally offer one or two years of pre-clinical study, often taught outside of the school and covering some or all, of the following courses:

- anatomy
- biomedical sciences
- physiology
- biochemistry
- oral biology
- pharmacology
- first aid
- introduction to the clinical skills that will be taught later in the course.

In addition, students will cover the effects of anaesthetics and other components common to medicine and dentistry. Furthermore, aspects of psychology will also be considered because dentists work in close proximity with people and use specific skills and techniques to relax patients.

Students who perform well in the examinations at the end of the pre-clinical course (year two) often take the opportunity to complete an intercalated BSc. This is normally a one-year project, during which students have the opportunity to investigate a chosen topic in much more depth, producing a written thesis before rejoining the course.

As the course progresses, the amount of clinical work that you carry out will increase, with most universities offering meaningful clinical contact from the third year. Alongside your clinical work, you will continue with programmes in areas such as oral biology, disease and pathology. You will also learn about the social and psychological aspects of patient care while developing your interpersonal and communication skills, and may be given the opportunity to spend some time in a general hospital.

As the clinical part of the course increases in importance, students often take responsibility for their own patients in the in-house 'mini-practices' or as part of a team comprising students with varied experience (in some schools, this includes training with chairside assistants, dental technicians and hygienists). During the clinical programme at Birmingham, for example, students are given responsibility for their own patients' treatment by what amounts to their own mini-practice in the dental hospital. Students are also encouraged to participate in practitioner attachment schemes in which they spend time with GDPs, specialist dental units and the SPCDS. Time can also be spent at local hospitals to gain experience of accident and emergency, ear, nose and throat, and general surgery. To teach the patient care necessary to effectively treat a range of people, many schools are now offering courses in behavioural sciences and the management of pain and anxiety, as well as in the treatment of children, the elderly and disabled people. The clinical students will typically study some of the following courses:

- behavioural science
- computing and statistics
- dental materials
- dental public health
- dental prosthetics
- haematology
- operative technique and clinical skills
- children's dentistry
- restorative dentistry
- oral medicine and surgery
- oral pathology
- oral biochemistry and biology
- orthodontics
- medico-legal and ethical aspects of dental practice
- forensic dentistry
- sedation
- radiology
- other aspects of the management of pain and anxiety in dentistry.

Your final year of study consists of a common core of academic work and clinical dental practice and is designed to consolidate and enhance all of the work and experience from your previous years of study. You will continue to have extensive and varied clinical exposure in a number of settings throughout this year. As you near the end of your clinical course, you are likely to have time to pursue your own elective programme of study – a topic of personal interest, which you research on your own. This elective study may include learning a foreign language and in some cases can involve travel abroad. For example, Cardiff is actively involved in the Erasmus exchange programme and has formal links with institutions in Sweden, the Netherlands, Italy and Turkey among others. Dundee also has links through the Erasmus programme with universities in Denmark, Finland, France, Germany and Norway. A number of other dental schools also have excellent working links with European universities. This means that under the Erasmus scheme, a limited number of students study at another participating European university and are accredited for the academic work they do there.

At the end of year five, there is the final BDS/BChD professional examination. On successful completion of the course, graduates are competent to carry out most treatments and exercise independent clinical judgement.

Two examples of course outlines are provided in the boxes below to illustrate the common threads and differences between different universities.

Programme structure - King's College London (2010)

'The King's dental degree programme, in line with General Dental Council recommendations, incorporates the latest thinking in dental education, early clinical exposure, an emphasis on ideas as well as facts, integrated teaching of all subjects with an emphasis on a systems approach, and a dimension of choice of special subjects by the student. The integrated nature of the programme means that basic science teaching will relate to clinical practice and clinical teaching will be underpinned by scientific understanding. You will have contact with patients from the first few weeks of the first year and will be encouraged to assume an appropriate level of responsibility for patient care at an early stage. The programme emphasises whole patient care, which implies consideration of the patient's total dental and medical needs, rather than just the provision of items of treatment. Most of the teaching is carried out in small groups where students and staff get to know each other well. The fact that the Dental Institute is the largest in the country with a total intake (for all programmes) of 164 students brings many advantages, including expertise in all areas of dentistry.

'The programme has three main components. The first consists of subjects common to medicine and dentistry, progressing from biomedical sciences, through behavioural sciences, epidemiology, pathology and microbiology to human disease. The second includes oral and dental aspects of the biological sciences leading to an understanding of the diagnosis, prevention and treatment of oral and dental diseases and disorders and the effects of systemic disease on the oral and dental tissues. The third component consists of the clinical and technical aspects of dentistry with the provision of comprehensive oral and dental healthcare for patients of all ages. These components are vertically integrated with a larger proportion of basic sciences at first and a larger clinical component at the end.

'Throughout the five years of the programme you will, in addition to acquiring the practical skills necessary to become a dentist, acquire communication skills, personal management skills, information technology skills and an appreciation and analysis of ethical and legal issues in dentistry.'

Source: www.kcl.ac.uk

Programme structure - University of Glasgow (2010)

'The current Glasgow BDS curriculum was introduced in 2004 and represents a radical change from the traditional dental programme. The biomedical and clinical medical sciences are taught in a completely integrated fashion with clinical dental sciences and communication skills, resulting in a truly student-centred learning experience.

'The early teaching of clinical dentistry is carried out in state-of-the-art clinical laboratories using simulated patient models. The clinical techniques laboratory and SimMan® patient simulator facility are enhancing significantly the educational experience of our dental undergraduates.

'Clinical teaching in the later years of the programme takes place in dental hospital clinics, which cover all the main specialities of restorative dentistry, oral surgery and oral medicine, paediatric dentistry, orthodontics and dental radiology. During the final year of the programme, you will spend 16 weeks in outreach clinics in primary care facilities with the Dental School, supervised by experienced dental surgeons.'

Source: www.gla.ac.uk

Postgraduate

There are many opportunities for postgraduate study in a variety of dental subjects. It is worth noting, however, that before any form of clinical training can commence (i.e. training involving hands-on contact with patients), dental graduates must register with the General Dental Council. Dental schools/hospitals run a wide range of postgraduate programmes that include further clinical and non-clinical training and research degree programmes. The postgraduate courses offered may be Diploma, Master or Doctorate and may take from one to two years, or in a few cases up to five years.

General advice and guidance are available from the Royal College of Surgeons of England (RCS) website (www.rcseng.ac.uk/fds/jcptd). However, the specific information related to each course is best obtained from the website or prospectus of the individual university; this will provide you with the most detailed, up-to-date information.

At Newcastle University, for example, there are four taught programmes. These are:

- Clinical Implant Training
- Diploma in Conscious Sedation

- Endodontics
- MSc in Restorative Dentistry.

Newcastle also offers research training that can lead to the degrees of MPhil, PhD or DDS. The MPhil normally requires 12 months' full-time or 24 months' part-time study; the PhD requires a minimum of 36 months' full-time study (most students complete this within four years); the DDS programmes are clinically based and generally take two to three years.

Other universities are also able to provide a wide range of postgraduate options. At King's College London for example, there are 17 taught graduate programmes, several of which can be pursued via distance learning.

As you might expect, there are also many openings for carrying out postgraduate research into related areas of dentistry at these institutions. However, both the taught and research postgraduate programmes can carry a premium that obviously intensifies if a candidate would like to pursue a doctorate.

In addition to the more formal postgraduate qualifications, qualified dentists are also required to participate in a specified amount of continuous professional development (CPD). This comprises courses for qualified dentists who want to develop their knowledge of the latest methods, equipment and techniques. Numerous institutions offer CPD, but there are details of a wide range of activities on each of the postgraduate deanery websites listed in Chapter 9.

Specialisms

The following sections briefly look at the major specialisations in dentistry.

Restorative dentistry

Restorative dentistry is the study, diagnosis and effective management of diseases of the teeth and their supporting structures. Restorative dentistry falls into three categories as described below.

1. Prosthodontics deals mainly with the replacement of hard and soft tissues using crowns, bridges, dentures and implants. It focuses on treatment planning, rehabilitation and maintenance of the oral function, comfort and appearance.
2. Periodontics is the branch of dentistry dealing with the supporting structures of teeth and includes the treatment of patients with severe gum disease.

3. Endodontics deals with health, injuries and diseases of the pulp and periradicular region (the tooth root and its surrounding tissue), such as root canal injuries, which can harm the nervous system as well.

Orthodontics

Orthodontics is a speciality of dentistry that is centred on the study and treatment of malocclusions (improper bites), which may result in tooth irregularity, out-of-proportion jaw relationships, or both. Orthodontic correction has a very positive effect on facial appearance.

Paediatric dentistry

Paediatric dentistry is the practice and teaching of and research into oral healthcare for children from birth to adolescence. Children are unique in their stages of development, oral disease and oral health needs, which is why paediatric dentistry covers all aspects of their oral healthcare. It aims to improve oral health in children and encourage the highest standards of clinical care. According to the BDA, research has shown that children who visit paediatric dentists are far less likely to require a repeat general anaesthetic for further dental treatment.

Oral surgery

Oral surgery is used to correct a wide spectrum of diseases, injuries and defects in the head, neck, face, jaws and the hard and soft tissues of the oral and maxillofacial region. It is a recognised international surgical speciality. Oral surgery is a slightly more intrusive form of surgery than typical root canal or cavity fillings. It usually requires the use of anaesthetic and therefore patients take longer to recover. Examples of oral surgery include having your wisdom teeth removed and getting dental implants.

Dental public health

Dental public health is a non-clinical speciality that includes assessment of dental health needs and ensuring that dental services meet those needs. It is mainly concerned with improving the dental health of a population rather than that of individuals and involves working in primary care trusts, government offices and strategic health authorities. There are a few such academic posts in universities and in the Department of Health.

Oral medicine

This is concerned with the diagnosis and non-surgical management of medical pathology affecting the oral area, jaw and face. Many oral medicine specialists have dual qualifications, with both medical and dental degrees. The main aspects of oral medicine are clinical care, research and undergraduate and postgraduate teaching.

Oral microbiology

This is the study of the diverse and complex microbial community in the mouth. Bacteria accumulate on both the hard and soft oral tissues. There is a highly developed defence system that monitors bacterial colonisation and prevents their invasion of local tissues.

Oral pathology

Oral pathology is the branch of dentistry concerned with diseases of oral structures, including soft tissues, teeth, jaws and salivary glands. Oral pathology is a science that investigates the causes, processes and effects of these diseases. The practice of oral pathology includes research and diagnosis of diseases using clinical, radiographic and biochemical means.

Forensic odontology

This is a relatively new and very exciting branch of dentistry and deals with the proper handling and examination of dental evidence, followed by its evaluation. It involves the identification of the causes of death or establishing vicinity and proof in a crime, for example, in the comparison of bite-marks on victims of assault and rape.

Dental and maxillofacial radiology

Dental and maxillofacial radiology involves a combination of radiology and dentistry. It is mainly concerned with using and understanding the diagnostic imaging modalities that are used in dentistry.

Prosthetics

Prosthetics is the science that is concerned with the diagnosis, prevention and treatment of disease of the teeth, gums, and related structures of the mouth, including the repair and replacement of defective teeth. The main areas that are covered by prosthetic dentistry are crowns (which provide full-coverage restoration of the tooth), bridges (which replace a missing tooth or teeth), dentures (which replace missing teeth or a full arch) and implants (which replace one or more missing teeth).

Cosmetic dentistry

The focal point of this type of dentistry involves improvements in appearance, either following trauma such as an accident or for perceived or real improvements in appearance to create a beautiful and healthy smile. This involves teeth whitening, tooth decorations (jewellery), cosmetic white fillings and cosmetic ceramic rims.

Fees and funding

Whether undertaking undergraduate or postgraduate studies, the costs can be considerable. A recent study involving 2,000 students found that students in England had an average debt of £5,293 per year; this means that, on average, a student completing a five-year dental course will accrue a debt of nearly £30,000. Bear in mind that this overall cost will fluctuate depending on a number of factors. Some of these are listed below.

- Geographical location – obviously studying in London is going to be more expensive than studying in Birmingham.
- Parental help – contributions from parents may significantly help meet the cost of living.
- Availability of scholarships – does the university offer scholarships for exceptional students?
- Finding a job – although it has the potential to interfere with you studies, working during your time at university will help to reduce the overall burden of debt.

Whatever the circumstances, you must give serious consideration to the cost and be prepared to commit fully for the duration of the course. To find out what the fees are and what funding is available for dentistry courses, you should explore each of the universities' websites and/or talk to their financial departments, because fees and funding procedures vary from university to university. You must also ensure that you plan your finances carefully in terms of tuition fees, living costs, and books and other necessary equipment. Needless to say living costs in big cities such as London will be much higher than in other parts of the country. One estimate suggests that it will cost up to £10,000 per year to cover your costs in London, significantly higher than the £5,293 national average figure quoted above.

Home students – that is UK nationals and EU students – pay lower tuition fees than non-EU/UK students. For the academic year 2010–11, the maximum tuition fees were £3,290, although you should expect this to rise. For international students from outside these two regions, the costs can be prohibitive. At Sheffield University, for example, the overseas tuition fees in 2010–11 are £14,380 per year for the first year and £25,900 for the remaining four years of the course.

Financial help

There are a number of sources of financial help that are potentially available for full-time students to help cover the cost of university study. The main ones are student grants, loans and bursaries, which are all allocated according to individual and family circumstances. It is important to apply as soon as possible through Student Finance England's online service (www.studentfinance.direct.gov)

Student grants

The Maintenance Grant is designed to help home students with accommodation and other living costs incurred while enrolled on a full-time course. These grants don't have to be repaid. If your family receives Income Support or another means-tested benefit, you may be eligible for the Special Support Grant instead of the Maintenance Grant.

The amount of grant a student receives depends on an assessment made by the local authority based on how much a student's parents earn. A student will only get a full grant if household income is judged to be £25,000 or less. Smaller amounts are available on a sliding scale, but any household with an income above £50,020 will not be eligible for any grant. An idea of the amount of grant awarded is given in Table 1.

Student loans

The most common way for students to finance their studies is by taking out a student loan. If you are an eligible, full-time student, you can take out two types of loan: a loan for tuition fees and a maintenance loan to meet living costs. The tuition fees loan does not depend on your household income and is paid straight to the university to cover the full cost.

The amount of maintenance loan you are entitled to depends on several factors, including household income, where you live while you're studying, when you started your course and whether you're in your final year. If you're living away from home, the maximum loan is £4,950 for the

Table 1 Amount of grant available based on family income 2010–11

Household income	Amount of grant for 2010–11
Up to £25,000	Full grant – £2,906
£30,000	£1,906
£34,000	£1,106
£40,000	£711
£45,000	£381
£50,020	£50
More than £50,020	No grant

See www.direct.gov.uk

academic year (2010–11) – more if you're studying in London. The maximum available is less if you're living with your parents during term time.

NHS bursaries

In 2010, NHS bursaries are expected to be available for full- and part-time students. To be eligible for such a bursary, a student must qualify as a home student and be on a course that is accepted as an NHS-funded place. These bursaries will be available for dentistry, as it is recognised as an NHS-funded course, but are not available during the first year of study. For more information, see the NHS students' bursaries website (www.nhsbsa.nhs.uk/Students/816.aspx).

Scholarships

Certain universities make scholarships available, and these can be a valuable source of income throughout a course. There are some general scholarships as well as ones available only to dentistry students. Details can be obtained from the individual universities, but websites such as www.scholarship-search.org.uk can provide comprehensive lists of available funding. In addition to this, the armed forces make scholarships available to students wishing to pursue a career in the medical services. These can be particularly lucrative and will often cover tuition fees as well as paying an annual salary for a part of the course. For example, some cadetships will pay all of your tuition fees, plus an annual salary for your last three years of study and a book allowance. Obviously, this route will not appeal to all students, as it guides you into a career in the armed forces.

For 2011–12 figures please check Student Finance England's website regularly.

3 | How do I complete my application and write an outstanding personal statement?

To gain a place at dental school, you have to submit a UCAS application. However, before you do so it is essential that you have thoroughly researched the application process and the demands of dentistry as a profession. Most people have little understanding of the tasks and challenges that a dentist faces on a day-to-day basis and the career pathways available after graduation. It is therefore vital that you are aware both of what being a dentist entails and of the details of the application process before you consider applying to study dentistry. This will ultimately mean that whatever choice you make it will be a well-informed one.

Choice of school

Once you have completed your work experience and are sure that you want to be a dentist, you need to research your choice of dental school.

There are various factors that you should take into account:

- the type and structure of the course
- the academic requirements
- whether the dental school requires you to sit the UKCAT
- location and type of university
- whether the dental school is part of a large university or a stand-alone medical and dental school.

The next step is to get hold of the prospectuses. If your school does not have spares, call the dental schools and they will send you copies free of charge. All universities offer detailed information on their websites, with some having complete online prospectuses, so it is well worth spending some time looking here as well. At the end of this book, there is a list of major dental organisations in the UK which you can contact for further information, and a list of the 14 dental schools and their contact details; you can approach the university with any questions relating to admissions or the course itself. What you must remember is that information on websites and in prospectuses is always changing, so if you're in doubt it is always best to call the university and speak to someone to get the most up-to-date information.

Once you have narrowed down the number of dental schools you like to, say, six or seven, you should try to visit them to get a better idea of what studying there will be like. Your school careers department will have details of open days (or you could call the dental schools directly), and some schools can arrange for you to be shown around at other times of the year as well. Do not simply select a dental school because someone has told you that it has a good reputation or that it is easier to get into. You will be spending the next five years of your life at one of them, and if you do not like the place you are unlikely to last the course.

Apart from talking to current or former dental students or careers advisers, there are a number of other sources of information that will help you in making your choice. The *Guardian* and *The Times* publish their own league tables of dental schools, ranked by a total score that combines several assessment categories, including teaching scores, student-staff ratios and job prospects. The 2010 *Guardian* table placed Birmingham first, followed by Dundee, Sheffield, Liverpool and Glasgow, while *The Times* placed Manchester first, followed by Sheffield, Glasgow, Birmingham, Newcastle and Dundee.

Of course, there is no such thing as a bad dental school in the UK, and league tables only tell you a small part of the whole story. They are based on a range of variables and this is why there is a discrepancy between the two newspapers' tables. Remember that league tables are only a guide – they are no substitute for visiting the dental schools, looking at the course content in detail, reading the prospectuses and speaking to those involved with the course.

Academic requirements

In addition to the grades they require at A level, all of the dental schools specify the minimum grades that they want at GCSE as well. This varies from dental school to dental school, but having at least five A or A* grades, with at least B grades in science subjects, English and mathematics is a significant advantage. There are some dental schools with lower requirements than others, so it is worth checking what each university is looking for. If your grades fall below these requirements, your referee will need to comment on them to explain why you underperformed (due to illness, family disruption etc.) and/or why they expect your A level performance to be better than your GCSE grades indicate.

If you are worried about achieving the right grades, you should think carefully about choosing at least two dental schools that accept retake candidates. Tables 2 and 3 in Chapter 9 give further information on this and show which dental schools consider students who have not achieved the minimum grades on their first attempt. The reason for including two (or more) of these dental schools is that many places will give preference to students who applied there the first time round. Some even specify it as a requirement for retakers.

In addition to specifying A level grades, some dental schools will ask for a minimum grade in the AS level subject you have studied. At the moment, some specify that this must be an A grade, others a B and others not at all. Perhaps even more important is the fact that AS levels contribute 50% to the total A level score, and poor AS level grades will make it difficult, if not impossible, to achieve A grades at A level. AS level grades also give admissions tutors more information to go on than GCSE grades and A level predictions alone, since the AS grades will be published in the August preceding your UCAS application. For the student, this means that the first year of A levels is just as important as the second.

The typical subject and entry grade requirements of each of the dental schools are shown in Tables 2 and 3 in Chapter 9. Also included in this table are details of GCSE and AS grade and subject requirements.

Another issue to be considered is the introduction of the A* grade at A level, as first awarded in August 2010. For entry in 2011, there are no dentistry courses that have made A* grades a part of their offers, and so at the moment there is no requirement to reach this level; however, it is probable that over the next few years offers for dentistry will include at least one A* grade.

Other qualifications

If you are not studying A levels, you should check with each dental school about their requirements. The list below offers a rough indication of what they might ask for.

- **Scottish Highers** – AAAAA–AAAAB at Higher level and two or three subjects at Advanced Higher. Higher level Chemistry and Biology are usually required, with at least one at Advanced Higher level.
- **International Baccalaureate** – 6/7, 6, 5/6 and 34–36 points overall. Chemistry and biology to be taken at Higher level, with passes in English and mathematics at Standard level.
- **European Baccalaureate** – 80%–85% overall, with 80% in each science option; chemistry and another science as full options.
- **Cambridge Pre-U** – most universities will accept Cambridge Pre-U qualifications with D3, D3, D3 in the principal subjects. Biology and chemistry will usually be required as two of the principal subjects.

- **Advanced diploma** – most universities do not accept the diploma for entry into dentistry; however, there are a few universities that will consider it alongside other qualifications. In these cases, it is best to contact the university directly to discuss entry requirements.
- **BTEC National Diploma** – some universities are happy to accept this with three Distinctions. However, most universities do not. Once again, it is best to contact the individual universities to discuss their entry requirements.

You will need to check with each university about their specific entry requirements as there is always some variation in their demands.

Non-dental choices

There are five spaces on the UCAS application, but only four of these can be used to select dentistry courses. Make sure you enter dentistry in all of the four spaces. The remaining space can be either left blank or filled with another course choice. Each university that you apply to will not see the other choices you have made and so you will not be discriminated against according to where else you have applied or what you have entered as your fifth choice. When filling in the final space, you must remember that it will have no impact on your other choices; however, you must also remember that you can only write one personal statement, which is likely to be largely irrelevant in relation to the other subject. So, for example, imagine you applied to four dental schools and then used your fifth space to apply for history. The dental schools you have chosen will not see that you have put history as your fifth choice and so this will not affect their judgement about your commitment to dentistry; however, the history admissions team will see from your personal statement that you are totally committed to dentistry and so are unlikely to make you an offer. In light of this, there are some subjects which are more appropriate to put as your fifth choice, such as dental hygiene and therapy or biomedical science, and you have a much greater chance of receiving an offer for one of these alongside an offer for dentistry. It can also provide you with another option to follow if you do not secure entry onto a dentistry course or do not achieve the necessary grades, keeping the door open for later graduate entry.

If you do decide to put another science-related course as your fifth choice, you still cannot make your personal statement relevant to more than one subject; keep it entirely focused on dentistry. Any attempt to make it attractive to a number of different admissions tutors in different subjects will adversely affect your chances of making a successful application to dentistry.

When thinking about which career to pursue, some students consider both dentistry and medicine at some point. If you consider applying for some dentistry and some medicine courses alongside each other, then you will be unsuccessful in securing a place on at least one of the subjects. You should make sure that you decide which path to follow as early as possible so that you can prepare the strongest possible application.

UKCAT

A number of dental schools now require applicants to sit the preadmissions test known as UKCAT (the UK Clinical Aptitude Test) before they apply. This test is designed to help discriminate between the many highly qualified applicants who apply for dentistry courses each year. It is important to note that the UKCAT is **not** based on science content from your A level science subjects, but on assessing your skills and attributes.

Dental schools currently requiring the test are Cardiff, Dundee, Glasgow, King's, Leeds, Manchester, Newcastle, Peninsula, Queen Mary, Queen's University Belfast and Sheffield.

Registration for the UKCAT usually opens in May of the year you submit your UCAS form and closes near the end of September. Testing then starts at the beginning of July and finishes at the start of October. It is vital to consult the UKCAT website (www.ukcat.ac.uk) for the exact registration and testing dates for the year you are applying, so that you know precisely what you need to do and when.

The first step is to register on the UKCAT website. You will be asked to select which test centre you wish to sit the test at and then the date and time. Registration opens in May and you should try to register as early as possible in order to get your preferred date and location; there are a number of students each year who have to travel great distances to find a test centre that still has spaces. It is worth taking the test as soon as possible so that you can make an informed decision about which universities to apply to. For example, if you apply only to universities that use the UKCAT and then you underperform in the test, it may reduce your chances of making a successful application. A much better route is to take the UKCAT before you finalise your choices; this will mean you can make a fully informed choice about which universities to apply to.

The cost for those who took the test in 2010 was £60 for candidates taking the test in the EU before 31 August and £95 for other candidates. Between 1 September and 10 October 2010, the cost was £75 for candidates taking the UKCAT in the EU. There are some bursaries available to students who may struggle to meet the cost of the test; these can be applied for through the UKCAT website.

The test itself is sat at an external centre in the location you have chosen. You should aim to arrive at least 15 minutes before your test time, remembering to take a printout of the email confirming your registration and photographic ID. It is important to remember that you must arrive on time for the slot you have booked; if you fail to do so, you will simply not be able to take the test and will have to rebook for a later date and pay the test fee again. The test lasts for two hours and consists of the following five sections:

I   verbal reasoning
2. quantitative reasoning
3. abstract reasoning
4. decision analysis
5. non-cognitive analysis.

Although the UKCAT website tries to discourage students from doing any preparation for the test, other than taking the practice test available on the website, students find that the more practice they have had on UKCAT-style questions, the better prepared they feel and the better they perform. There are numerous books available that offer hints, tips and practice questions; it is worth flicking through the various titles in a bookshop to see which is best suited to your needs.

The structure and layout of each section is described below.

1. Verbal reasoning

This section is 22 minutes long and contains 44 questions. The UKCAT website says that this section 'assesses candidates' ability to think logically about written information and to arrive at a reasoned conclusion.'

You will be presented a short passage of text (an example is given in Figure 1) and given four statements relating to each passage.

UKCAT Practice Test 3 (Short Version)

In digital recording, the analogue sound that we hear needs to be translated into a series of numbers ('0' or '1'). These numbers represent the changes in air pressure over time that make up the sound, though we cannot directly 'hear' these numbers as sound.

Digital recordings are made by sending the original analogue sound to an 'analogue to digital converter' (ADC). This converter changes the analogue signal into a series of binary numbers. These numbers are then usually stored on a computer or a compact disc. During playback, the digital sound information is read and sent to a 'digital to analogue converter' (DAC) which changes the sound into an analogue signal that is reproduced by devices such as a loudspeaker or headphones.

Figure 1 Sample UKCAT verbal reasoning passage

For each statement, you must answer 'true', 'false' or 'can't tell' based on the information you are given in the passage (see Figure 2).

A loudspeaker is able to produce an analogue signal.

A. True

B. False

C. Can't tell

Figure 2 Sample UKCAT verbal reasoning question

There are 11 passages in this section, giving 44 questions in total.

2. Quantitative reasoning

This section is 23 minutes long and contains 44 questions. The UKCAT website says that it 'assesses candidates' ability to solve numerical problems.'

In this section, you will be presented with some numerical data and then be asked to answer four related questions. Each question has five possible answers to choose from, as shown in Figures 3 and 4.

A distribution centre serves stores within a 50 mile radius. The table below shows how far each store is from the distribution centre.

Distance from distribution centre	Number of stores
10 miles or less	3
11 to 20 miles	15
21 to 30 miles	26
31 to 40 miles	20
41 to 50 miles	16

Figure 3 Sample UKCAT numerical data table

How many stores does the distribution centre serve?

A. 60

B. 70

C. 80

D. 90

E. Can't tell

Figure 4 Sample UKCAT numerical data table

There are 11 sets of data, giving 44 questions in total.

3. Abstract reasoning

This section is 16 minutes long and contains 65 questions. The UKCAT website says that it 'assesses candidates' ability to infer relationships from information by convergent and divergent thinking.'

In this section you will be presented with two sets of shapes, set A and B, as in Figure 5.

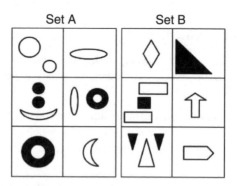

Figure 5 Sample UKCAT shape sets

For each pair of set A and B, you will be presented with five test shapes, as in Figure 6.

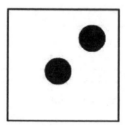

A. Set A

B. Set B

C. Neither

Figure 6 Sample UKCAT test shapes

With each shape, you have to decide whether they belong to set A, set B or to neither. There are 13 sets of A and B giving 65 questions in total.

4. Decision analysis

This section is 32 minutes long and contains 28 items. The UKCAT website says that it 'assesses candidates' ability to deal with various forms of information, to infer relationships, to make informed judgements, and to decide on an appropriate response in situations of complexity and ambiguity.'

In this section you will be presented with a table of codes, as for example in Figure 7.

Additional codes

Operators General Rules	Specific Info Basic Codes	Complex Info Additional Information	Reactions/ Outcomes Emotions
A = positive	1 = personal	101 = speed	201 = hurt
B = increase	2 = people	102 = injury	202 = excited
C = opposite	3 = air	103 = danger	203 = worried
D = cold	4 = fire	104 = fun	204 = angry
E = fast	5 = water	105 = carry	205 = surprise
F = generalise	6 = earth	106 = empty	
G = combine	7 = sun		
	8 = moon		
	9 = dwelling		
	10 = move		
	11 = today		
	12 = light		
	13 = bag		
	14 = look		

Figure 7 Sample UKCAT decision analysis code table

You will then be presented with 26 questions related to this table that will require you to decode or encode information or decide on the most appropriate words to add to the table of codes. Each question will have four or five possible answer choices, as shown in Figure 8, for example.

5. Non-cognitive analysis

This section is 27 minutes long. The UKCAT website says that it 'identifies the attributes and characteristics of robustness, empathy and integrity that may contribute to successful health professional practice.'

What is the best interpretation of the following coded message:

11, 12, 7

A. Today it is bright and sunny

B. The light from the sun is brighter than usual

C. Today the sun came up

D. Today the sun's rays have a strange hue

E. The sun is floating in the sky

Figure 8 Sample UKCAT decision analysis answer choices

All sample UKCAT questions reprinted with kind permission of UKCAT and Pearson VUE.

Currently, the responses from this section of the test are not used in the selection process.

The biggest challenge you will face while taking the test is lack of time because there are so many questions to answer in such a short period. It is vital for you to use the practice tests to get a feel for what it is like to be in a time-pressured situation and to understand how long you can spend on each question in each section.

Personal statement

As has been previously stated, the number of candidates applying for dentistry courses has seen a steady increase over recent years and is expected to continue rising. So what exactly does this rise in applicants for dentistry mean?

Almost certainly, the grades necessary for entry into dental school will continue to rise, and in order to differentiate between applicants universities will set very high entry requirements. In the late 1990s, when application numbers were lower, candidates often received BBC offers, whereas now the standard offer is likely to be AAB or AAA and if you are a retake candidate then you are most likely to be asked for AAA. At some point in the future, a standard offer is likely to include at least one A* at A level as well.

As a consequence of the increasing number of applicants, your application is likely to be received by the university and considered along with many others at the same time. On average, a dental school may receive around 700 applications and have to select around 250–300 to be called for interview. Of those who apply, there will be some who are automatically rejected as they do not fulfil all the entry criteria; for example, not meeting the GCSE grade requirements. Following this, it is down to the admissions team to try to select whom to interview from the remaining candidates. Many of the applicants who are still being considered at this stage will have excellent GCSE profiles, outstanding predicted A level grades and a strong UKCAT performance. So how do the selectors make their choices?

One of the most important factors in this stage of selection is the personal statement. If this is badly worded, uninteresting or lacking the things that the selector feels are important, it will be put on the 'reject without interview' pile. Ultimately, this means that the more thought that you give to your UCAS application and personal statement, the better it will be and the greater your chance of being offered a conditional place or being asked to come in for an interview. Remember that the selectors will not know about the things that you have forgotten to say: they can only get an impression of you from what is in the application. I have come across many good students who never secured an interview simply because they did not thoroughly plan and prepare their personal statement.

Note that only a small proportion of applicants will be interviewed. The number of those interviewed depends on the university. Tables 2 and 3 in Chapter 9 provide an outline of the percentage and numbers in real terms that dental schools interview. For example, the interview policy at Liverpool is to see around 40% of those who apply, which for 2010 entry meant 358 interviews out of 883 applications.

All applicants now submit their applications via Apply on www.ucas.ac.uk; follow the instructions and use the drop-down menus and 'help' features to avoid errors. Also ensure that you make use of the advice and guidance available at your school or college, as this will help you avoid common mistakes. Once you have completed and submitted your application, it is automatically passed to your referee, who will enter your reference then submit it to UCAS.

The following sections will tell you more about what the selectors are looking for in a personal statement, and how you can avoid common mistakes.

When constructing your personal statement, there are several important things that you need to consider. First, your personal statement needs to be no more than 47 lines or 4,000 characters including spaces; this is a strict limit and so you need to ensure that you are as close to this as possible. You must then consider the key themes of your personal statement, which are:

- why you want to be a dentist
- what your academic interests are and how these have furthered your desire to pursue dentistry

- what you have done to investigate the profession
- what you have done to develop the skills needed to become a dentist
- why you are the right person for their dental school and their particular dentistry course.

The personal statement is your opportunity to demonstrate to the selectors that you are fully committed to studying dentistry and have the right motivation and personal qualities to do so successfully. Do not be tempted to write the statement in the sort of formal English that you find in, for example, job applications. Read through a draft of your statement, and ask yourself the question 'Does it sound like me?' If not, rewrite it. For example, avoid phrases such as 'I was fortunate enough to be able to shadow a dentist . . .' when you really just mean 'I shadowed a dentist . . .' or 'I arranged to shadow a dentist . . .'.

Why dentistry?

A high proportion of UCAS applications contain stock phrases such as: 'From an early age I have wanted to be a dentist because it is the only career that combines my love of science with the chance to work with people.' Not only do admissions tutors get bored with reading such statements, remarks like these are also clearly untrue: if you think about it, there are many careers that combine science and working with people, including teaching, pharmacy, physiotherapy and nursing. Nevertheless, the basic idea of this sentence may well apply to you. If so, you need to personalise it. You could mention an incident that first got you interested in dentistry – a visit to your own dentist, a conversation with a family friend or a talk or lesson at school, for instance. You could write about your interest in human biology or a biology project that you did when you were younger to illustrate your interest in science, and then give examples of how you like to work with others. You should also ensure that you avoid giving reasons relating to money or status; any mention of wanting to be a dentist so that you can earn £200,000 a year is an almost guaranteed way of being rejected!

Your academic interests

It is important for your personal statement to contain information about your academic interests and how they have furthered your desire to study dentistry. This may be related to some topics or practical skills that have been of particular interest to you over the course of your studies, or to an interesting article you have read in a newspaper or journal, or to something engaging you heard at a lecture. Whatever it is, it will help to demonstrate your desire to pursue the course, as long as you make it relevant to dentistry.

It is then important to back up evidence of your initial interest in dentistry with details of what you have done to investigate the career.

What have you done to research dentistry?

This is where you can describe your work experience. It is important to demonstrate that you gained something from the work experience, and that it has given you an insight into the profession. You should give an indication of the length of time you spent at each dental practice, what treatments you observed, and the impressions you've gained of dentistry. You could comment on what aspects of dentistry attract you, what you found interesting or something that you hadn't expected. Beyond this, you should also make mention of any other work experience you have had in a caring or clinical role and what you learned from it. Although you may not think of these sorts of experiences as being relevant, they can often demonstrate to an admissions tutor good interpersonal skills or commitment and dedication, all of which are relevant to dentistry.

Here is a sample description of a student's work experience that would probably not impress the admissions team.

> 'I spent three days at my local dental practice. I saw some patients having fillings, and a man whose false teeth didn't fit. It was very interesting.'

In contrast, the example below would be much more convincing because it is clear that the student is interested in what was happening.

> 'During my two weeks at the Smith and Smith Dental Clinic, I shadowed two dentists and a hygienist. I watched a range of treatments including fillings, a root canal, extractions and orthodontic treatment. I found particularly interesting the fact that, although both dentists had very different personalities, they both related well to the patients, who seemed to find them very reassuring. A number of things surprised me; in particular, how demanding a dentist's day is.'

It will be far easier to write this section of your personal statement if you spent some time making notes during your work experience. Look back over what you wrote and use your thoughts and experiences as a stimulus for this section. With luck, the selectors will pick up on these experiences at interview and ask you to expand on some of your comments. They may ask questions about the methods that the dentists used to relax their patients, or what you perceived the demands of dentistry to be.

Evidence of developing skills and personal qualities

As a dentist, you will be working with a wide range of professionals and patients throughout your career. To qualify as a dentist, you will study alongside possibly 50 other students in your year, for five years. The person reading your UCAS application has to decide two things: whether you have the right skills and personal qualities to become a successful dentist, and whether you will be able to cope with and contribute to dental school life. To be a successful dentist, you need (among other things!) to:

- be able to survive and enjoy dental school
- have good interpersonal skills and get on with a wide range of people
- be able to work under pressure and cope with stress
- have well-developed manual skills.

How, then, does the person reading your personal statement know whether you have the qualities they are looking for? What you must remember is that the admissions tutor doesn't know you, so you should give lots of evidence of how you have demonstrated and developed these qualities. Some of the things they may be looking for are:

- participation in team events
- involvement in school plays or concerts
- positions of responsibility
- work in the local community
- part-time or holiday jobs
- an ability to get on with people
- participation in activities involving manual dexterity.

What they don't want to hear is how you have demonstrated interpersonal skills by going into town every weekend or how you have improved your manual dexterity by playing PlayStation 3 games!

The selectors will be aware that some schools offer more to their students in the way of activities and responsibilities than others. However, even if there are very few opportunities made available to you through your school, you must still find ways to gain experience and develop your skills. You don't have to have been captain of the rugby team or gone on a three-month expedition to Borneo to be considered, but you do need to be able to demonstrate that you have made efforts to participate in a range of worthwhile activities.

Remember, however, that while evidence of all these skills and extra interests is extremely important, it will not compensate for lower grades, so having a strong academic profile and getting high grades still remains the most important aspect of your application.

Weak and strong personal statements – exemplars

The box below gives an example of a personal statement I have constructed based on experience of reading through what students write. It is made up of a combination of some good ideas, points that need to be expanded on and things not to say! Overall, as you will probably notice, this would be considered as a weak statement and be unlikely to lead to an offer being made.

DO NOT COPY ANY PARTS OF THESE PERSONAL STATEMENTS!

You should use these examples to give you an idea of structure and the type of content you may want to include, but universities have sophisticated software to detect copied parts of personal statements so do not be tempted! Your personal statement should be personal to you and above all else it should be honest.

Personal statement: Example 1 (character count: 1,552)

I originally wanted to study medicine, but thought being a doctor was very difficult, so I decided to change my mind and study dentistry. I really enjoy working with people and have always enjoyed studying science at school so I think dentistry would be ideal for me. I also feel that I work well on my own but can also work well in a team. My motivation to study dentistry comes from seeing my uncle work as a dentist and also seeing how much money he earns. I would ultimately like to pursue a career as a cosmetic dentist.

During the Easter holiday, I spent three weeks shadowing a general dental practitioner at my local dental practice. I really enjoyed watching the dentist work and gained a real insight into the skills needed to be a dentist. I also try to keep up to date with the latest developments in dentistry by reading news and journal articles. At the moment I am studying Biology, Chemistry and Psychology at A level. I really enjoy my subjects and feel they will provide me with knowledge and understanding that is particularly appropriate to studying dentistry. I feel that carrying out practical work in biology and chemistry has helped me to develop my manual dexterity skills.

I also have a number of interests outside of school. I like relaxing and enjoy watching TV. I also like going out with my mates at the weekend. I play football in a local league, read science fiction

---

> books, play the piano, go to the gym and listen to music. I also have a Saturday job which gives me some extra money to spend when I go out with my mates.

Personal statement: Example 1 raises a number of interesting points.

1. It is too short.

This statement is just over 1,500 characters. The limit is 4,000 characters (including spaces) and you should aim to use as much of this as possible.

- *It lacks detail and specific examples.*

  The candidate has got the right idea about the structure and addressed the key sections. However, it is very light on actual detail and doesn't really expand on any of the points made or give specific examples. When discussing work experience, go into detail about what you witnessed and what you learned. When giving details of what you are studying, be specific about topics you have enjoyed. This will give the admissions tutor a much greater insight into who you are and the skills you possess.

- *It is not very personal.*

  This could be about any number of candidates applying to dentistry. Make sure your personal statement has evidence and experiences to show an admissions tutor who you really are.

2. Never start with a negative.

I have seen many personal statements start on a negative point, as is the case here. Any negative points – for example, about things you don't like – do not need to be included. The overall tone should be optimistic and positive.

- *Money should not be your main motivation.*

  Although most dentistry applicants will have thought about how much money they will be making at some point, it is not something that needs to be highlighted in your personal statement. Your reasons for studying dentistry need to run much deeper than this if you are going to get into dental school.

- *Dentistry is more than cosmetic enhancements.*

  Lots of people fixate on the idea of specialising in cosmetic dentistry. However, dentistry is a far broader discipline and a personal statement should really reflect an understanding of this fact.

- *Practical work is not the only way of demonstrating manual dexterity.*

  If you are going to use the example of science practicals to demonstrate your manual dexterity, give specific examples of those you have enjoyed or apparatus you have used. You must also try to think of other activities that have helped you demonstrate these skills.

- *Avoid lists of interests.*
  It can be very easy to simply reduce your extracurricular activities into a long list. Take time to explain what you gain from each of your interests and how they benefit your application. In addition to this, avoid mentioning mundane interests such as going out with friends and watching TV, because they tell the admissions tutor very little about you.

Although this statement is poor, it would not need much effort to make it a reasonable attempt, as the basic structure is fine. Your first attempt at writing a personal statement will probably be difficult and might not produce great results; however, it is important that you get feedback on your efforts and then redraft it as many times as necessary. The best personal statements can take up to 10 drafts to get completely right! Some changes that would be worth making are shown in the following box.

I originally wanted to study medicine, but thought being a doctor was very difficult, so I decided to change my mind and study dentistry. [*Remove this and try to start on a positive*] I really enjoy working with people [*Give examples of where you have done this*] and have always enjoyed studying science at school so I think dentistry would be ideal for me. I also feel that I work well on my own but can also work well in a team. [*Again, give examples*] My motivation to study dentistry comes from seeing my uncle work as a dentist and also seeing how much money he earns. [*Remove the reference to money*] I would ultimately like to pursue a career as a cosmetic dentist. [*Explain why*]

During the Easter holiday, I spent three weeks shadowing a general dental practitioner at my local dental practice. I really enjoyed watching the dentist work and gained a real insight into the skills needed to be a dentist. [*What exactly did you observe, what did you learn, what interested you?*] I also try to keep up to date with the latest developments in dentistry by reading news and journal articles. [*What have you read about and what topics particularly interest you?*] At the moment I am studying Biology, Chemistry and Psychology at A level. I really enjoy my subjects and feel they will provide me with knowledge and understanding that is particularly appropriate to studying dentistry. [*Be specific about which topics you have enjoyed studying and why they are of interest to you*] I feel that carrying out practical work in biology and chemistry has helped me to develop my manual dexterity skills. [*Which practicals have you enjoyed?*]

I also have a number of interests outside of school. I like relaxing and enjoy watching TV. I also like going out with my mates at the weekend. [*Be imaginative! Nobody is particularly interested in this!*] I play football in a local league, read science fiction books, play the piano, go to the gym and listen to music. I also have a Saturday job which gives me some extra money to spend when I go out with my mates. [*Try to avoid long lists of interests – you will do much better to expand on the really interesting ones; for example, playing piano is the most important here as it demonstrates manual dexterity*]

Here are two examples of much better personal statements based on those written by two students who both secured entry onto dental courses. Each demonstrates clarity and focus, and what comes through is the enthusiasm that the candidates have for dentistry.

Personal statement: Example 2 (character count: 2,867)

While volunteering in China I was compelled to reflect on the importance of dental care in all our lives. I worked with disabled orphans, many of whom suffered from dental-related pain. It was a humbling experience that made me appreciate the level of dental care I received at home, and how I had taken it for granted. I began research into dentistry and organised several sessions of work experience, giving me a clearer understanding of the everyday demands that dentists face. I am drawn to a career which helps people, allows me to build on my appetite for scientific understanding, and to implement that understanding in a practical way.

I shadowed dentists in general and community dental practices, witnessing simple and restorative treatments; my experiences taught me the importance of good communication skills and the flexibility needed in a surgery. To build on these observations I secured work as a dental receptionist and exercised the skills needed to work with demanding patients. The position required me to work quickly and accurately. These skills were tested in my involvement in the launch of a dental practitioners accreditation scheme while working as part of the Heart of Birmingham PCT. The aim of the initiative was to encourage implementation of the clinical governance framework to improve levels of customer service in practices.

Volunteering for Dent-Aid enhanced my proficiency as a public speaker and inspired me to work with vulnerable people by carrying out voluntary work for St John Ambulance. As a first-aider, I had the experience of dealing with people with low self-esteem and communication problems; both of these experiences have relevance to becoming a successful dentist and highlighted the importance of empathy when dealing with patients.

At my school, my position as vice house captain was to lead and motivate the house to work together as a team, highlighting both my ability to handle responsibility and leadership skills. Being charity prefect and maths mentor developed my skills in forming relationships, an ability I hope I can transfer to the dental profession. Completing the Duke of Edinburgh's Gold Award furthered my leadership and teamwork skills; I tackled the difficulties we faced with a logical outlook. My determination and persistence are also shown through my achieving 1st and 2nd Dan black belts in Karate, and in swimming, in which I have gained gold and honours awards. I achieved 91/95 in my GCSE textiles coursework and my interest in sewing remains as I continue to personalise my wardrobe. My precision and steady hand give me the physical skills needed for a prospective dental student.

I believe that the range of skills I have acquired from my school life and extracurricular activities, as well as my hard-working nature, gives me the potential to flourish as a member of the dental profession.

Personal statement: Example 2, although lacking in some areas, gives a real impression of dedication to pursuing dentistry and demonstrates a very clear and believable explanation of why this student wants to pursue dentistry. They have lots of relevant work experience and really make the most of expanding on what they have learned from it. In addition, this student has really picked out the key extracurricular activities and elaborated on their importance. The small weaknesses are that it doesn't really deal with academic areas of interest and doesn't have too much to say about developing manual dexterity.

Personal statement: Example 3 (character count: 3,695)

My passion to study dentistry has been reinforced by the many hours of work experience I have undertaken. Every time I have had the chance to observe a dentist, I have been amazed by the different skills and level of technical ability required. I have also been able to identify the importance of the dentist–patient relationship and the need for having empathy and well-developed communication skills. What really intrigued me was that even though the procedures are the same, no two mouths are. This gave me the inspiration to look into the profession in greater detail.

During my two-month placement at Aesthetics dental practice, I shadowed two dentists, a dental technician and a dental hygienist. This allowed me to see the intricate workings of a practice from different levels of the organisation and appreciate the importance of teamwork and co-operation within the surgery. I was also fortunate enough to see a wide range of treatments, ranging from fillings to root canals. To further my knowledge of dentistry, I attended a dental day at the University of London. I met many people from different fields, including a paediatric dentist and a maxillofacial surgeon. After two weeks of work experience in a primary school I decided I would very much like to work in the field of paediatric dentistry in order to give children positive experiences of visiting the dentist and promote good oral health.

Studying biology and chemistry at A level has been challenging and encourages me to pursue this career. My practical work in biology and chemistry provides an excellent opportunity to work with my hands and gives me an opportunity to observe how the theory and practical work are interrelated. I particularly enjoyed carrying out practicals related to measuring enzyme activity and also the intricate nature of titrations. I also thoroughly enjoyed studying diseases such as TB and cholera, which led me to research diseases in the dental field such as gingivitis and dry mouth. Chemistry has been a particularly rewarding subject; I particularly enjoyed learning the different mechanisms in organic chemistry and carrying out complex calculations.

Over the past six months I have carried out voluntary work at a local hospice. This has enabled me to meet and relate to a variety of different people from many diverse backgrounds. Working in a caring environment has shown me the meaning of empathy and working with fragile people. One of the most important lessons I have learned is that patients can often be fragile and patience is vital. Knowing that I had contributed to making somebody's quality of life better has influenced my enthusiasm to study dentistry, as I feel that I can continue to do this by pursing dentistry as a career.

In Year 11, I was appointed Head Boy at my school. My responsibilities included delivering speeches, representing the school at numerous events and working as part of a team with the house captains and deputies to organise fund-raising events. Altogether we managed to raise £1,057. I also have a keen interest in making and painting model aeroplanes and cars and have been doing so since I was young. This has given me excellent fine motor skills and has taught me how to manipulate very small pieces of equipment in very confined spaces; all of which is directly relevant to being a dentist.

I know that dentistry is demanding and challenging, but I feel I have all of the necessary attributes to become a first-class dentist. I am a very determined person and this is why I am committed to succeed. I adopt a 'do not give up' policy in my life and I feel this has been shown by the many different areas that I have participated and had success in.

Personal statement: Example 3 has a number of very strong points. The point of a personal statement is that it should be personal and reflect as much as possible a candidate's individuality; I feel that this statement does this well. It also makes clear the academic interests that the student has and how they link in to studying dentistry. It also deals with manual dexterity very clearly. I think the strongest feature here is that it demonstrates a high degree of selflessness and care for others; this is shown through the examples of voluntary work carried out. I certainly get the feeling that this student is genuinely interested in pursuing this career path for the right reasons.

The reference

As well as your GCSE results and your personal statement, the admissions team will take into account your academic reference. This is where your headmaster or headmistress, housemaster or housemistress or head of sixth form writes about what an outstanding person you are, how you are the life and soul of the school, how you are on target for three A grades at A level and why you will become an outstanding dentist. For him or her to say this, of course, it has to be true. The referee is expected to be as honest as possible, and to try to accurately assess your character and potential. You may believe that you have all of the qualities – academic and personal – necessary in a dentist, but unless you have demonstrated these to your teachers, they will be unable to support your application.

Ideally, your efforts to impress them will have begun at the start of the sixth form (or preferably before this): you will have become involved in school activities, while at the same time working hard in your A level subjects and developing strong interpersonal skills, demonstrated by your interactions with staff and students. If you do not feel as though you have done this, don't worry, because it is never too late. Some people mature later than others, so if this does not sound like you, start to make efforts to get involved in the wider life of your school or college, as this will help to give evidence to the people who will contribute to your reference.

As part of the reference, your referee will need to predict the grades that you are likely to achieve. As Table 2 in Chapter 9 (page 108) shows, the minimum requirement is AAB. If you are predicted lower than this, it is unlikely that you will be considered. Talk to your teachers and find out whether you are on target for these grades. If not, you need to do one or all of the following:

- work harder or more effectively – and make sure that your teachers notice that you are doing so
- get some extra help either at school or outside – for instance an Easter revision course
- delay submitting your UCAS application until you have your A level results.

When to submit the UCAS application

The closing date for receipt of the application by UCAS is 15 October. However, you must remember that this is the deadline by which the form is required by UCAS and so your school or college will most likely have an earlier deadline so they can get your reference written. This will probably be around two weeks earlier. Late applications are accepted by UCAS, but the dental schools are not obliged to consider them; because of the pressure on places, it is unlikely that late applications will be considered. Although you can submit your application any time between the beginning of September and the October deadline, most admissions tutors agree that the earlier the application is submitted, the better your chance of being called for interview.

The safest bet for getting your application completed and sent as soon as possible is to make a start on it in your AS year. Start researching the different universities and the different courses as soon as possible and then begin writing your personal statement and get feedback on it. Ultimately, you want to be in a position where you have a final draft of your personal statement and all of your choices sorted by the beginning of the September term in your A2 year.

Checklist

- Do you have at least two weeks' work-shadowing experience?
- Do you meet the GCSE requirements for your chosen universities?
- Are you on target for at least AAB?
- Have you researched the different dental schools and their courses?
- Have you been to university open days?
- Have you completed the UKCAT?
- Does your personal statement demonstrate commitment, research, personal qualities, communication skills and manual dexterity?

Deferred entry

Most admissions tutors are happy to consider students who take a gap year, and many encourage it. However, if you are considering a gap year, you need to make sure that you are going to use the time constructively. A year spent watching daytime TV is not going to impress anybody, whereas independent travelling, charity or voluntary work either at home or abroad, work experience or a responsible job will all indicate that you have used the time to develop independence and maturity.

Having a job during your gap year in somewhere like a shop or a bar may seem like a good idea and is certainly better than sitting around doing nothing all the time; however, if you wish to demonstrate your ongoing commitment to pursuing dentistry as a career, then you should concentrate on getting further experience in a job or placement directly related to the field.

You can either apply for deferred entry when you submit your UCAS application, in which case you need to outline your plans clearly in your personal statement, or apply in September following the publication of your A level results. If you expect to be predicted the right grades, and the feedback from your school or college is that you will be given a good reference, you should apply for deferred entry; but if you are advised by your referee that you are unlikely to be considered, you should give yourself more time to work with your referees by waiting until you have your A level results.

What happens next?

About a week after UCAS receives your application, it will send you a welcome letter and an applicant welcome guide, confirming your personal details and choices. It is vital that you check this information carefully and inform UCAS if there are any inaccuracies. A common mistake is to select the foundation year – the 'pre-dental' year – rather than the start of the course proper, so make sure you haven't done this. Remember, you will be able to access your application at all times through the UCAS Track system using the same personal ID, user-name and password that you used to apply.

As soon as UCAS processes your application, your prospective universities can access it, but they will be unable to see the other courses and universities that you have applied to. Once a university has accessed your application, they may contact you to acknowledge receipt of your application; however, not all universities bother doing this, so don't worry if you don't hear from them initially.

The next stage is to wait to hear from the universities you applied to, once they have considered your application. If you are lucky, you will hear from the dental schools asking you to attend an interview. Some dental schools interview on a first come, first served basis, while others wait until all applications are in before deciding whom to interview. It is not uncommon for students to hear nothing until after Christmas, so don't panic if you aren't contacted straight away.

If you are unlucky, you will receive a notification from UCAS telling you that you have been rejected by one or more of the dental schools. If this happens, don't despair: you may hear better news from another of the schools that you applied to. If you end up with four rejections, you should take the opportunity to carefully reassess whether dentistry is a realistic career ambition for you and whether there were any parts of your application that let you down. If you still feel that dentistry is for you, take the opportunity to strengthen any aspects of your application that were weak. Under no circumstances should you give up and decide that it is no longer worth working hard; this will only reduce your chances of making a successful application the following year.

Note that going through Clearing in August is no longer an option for entry into dentistry. Places are limited and often oversubscribed, and more offers are made than there are places available. There can be the odd exception on a year-to-year basis where a few places are available; however, under no circumstances should you bank on any such places becoming available.

Dental timeline

Figure 9 shows the tasks that you will need to be aware of over the course of your A level studies and gives an overview of the timing of some of the various tasks that you should plan for if you are to maximise your chances of gaining entry into a dental school.

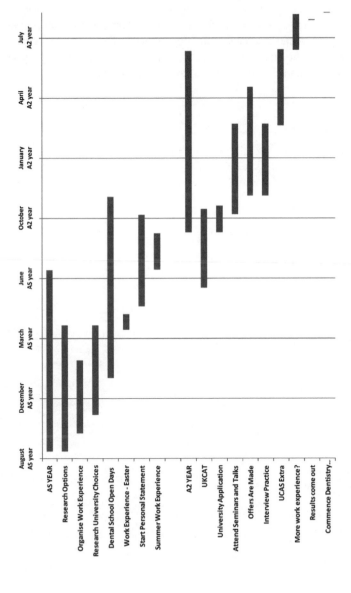

Figure 9 Timeline to guide your application to study dentistry

As you can see, your main task in your AS year is to start researching your courses and options, organising and carrying out work experience and then preparing your personal statement. The summer between your AS and A2 years should be used to continue building your work experience as well as registering and preparing for UKCAT. In the second year you must hit the ground running, because UKCAT and your UCAS application must be finished by early October. At the same time, you must also ensure that you stay on top of your studies so you maximise your chances of achieving the A grades you will need, and you should also start preparing for interview and practising your interview skills. Once your final exams are finished at the end of the year, it is simply a matter of waiting for your results so you can see whether you have secured a place.

4 | What makes a successful interview?

Once you've submitted your UCAS application, you must wait to hear from each of the universities you have applied to. If you meet their entry criteria and they like the look of your application, they will probably call you for interview. The universities use interviews to find out first-hand whether the picture painted by your application is accurate and to investigate your suitability for their course. The questions asked of you in an interview will generally be designed to:

- relax you – interviewers wish to see the real you and this will come across more clearly if you are relaxed
- investigate your interest in and suitability for dentistry
- get a clearer picture of your personal qualities.

Questions to get you relaxed

Question: How was your journey here today?

Comment: The interviewers are not really interested in the details of your journey. Do not be tempted to give them a minute-by-minute account of your bus journey or to simply say 'OK'. You should give a answer that is honest and fairly brief; maybe giving them an idea of where you came from and how long the journey took, or give them details of some relevant reading or preparation you did on the journey.

Question: Tell me why you decided to apply to Shufflefield.

Comment: Another variation on this might be: 'How did you narrow your choice down to four dental schools?' The panel will be looking for evidence of research, and that your reasons are based on informed judgement. Probably the best possible answer would start with 'I came to your open day . . .' because you can then proceed to tell them why you like their university so much, what impressed you about the course and facilities and how the atmosphere of the place would particularly suit you. If you are/were unable to attend open days, try to arrange a formal or informal visit before you are interviewed so that you can show that you are aware of the environment, both academic and physical, and that you like the place. If you know people who are at the dental school or university, so much the better. You should also know about the course structure: the prospectus will give detailed information. Given the choice between a candidate who is not only going to make a good dentist but clearly wants to come to their institution, and another who may have the right qualities but does not seem to care whether it is there or somewhere else that they study, who do you think the selectors will choose?

Answers to avoid are ones such as 'Reputation' (unless you know in detail the areas for which the dental school is highly regarded), 'I don't want to move away from my friends', 'You take a lot of retake students' or 'My dad says it's easy to get a place here'.

It is vital to do your homework by reading the prospectus and looking at the website. Although on the surface all dental courses appear to cover broadly the same subjects, there are big differences between the ways courses are delivered and in the opportunities for patient contact, and your interviewers will expect you to know about their course. A good answer could be 'I came to an open day last summer, which is why I have applied here. I enjoyed the day, and was impressed by the facilities and the comments of the students who showed us around, because they seemed so enthusiastic about the course. Also, I really like the emphasis that the course has on early clinical contact.' There are many variations on this question, so take time to reflect on your own personal reasons.

The interviewers may ask you what you know about the course, or about the dental school. In all cases, this is your chance to show the interviewers that you are desperate to come to their institution.

Questions about dentistry

Question: Why do you want to be a dentist?

Comment: This is the question that all interviewees expect. Given that the interviewers will be aware that you are expecting the question, they will also expect your answer to be carefully planned. If you look surprised and say something like 'Um . . . well . . . I haven't really thought about why . . .' you can expect to be rejected. Other answers to avoid are those along the lines of 'The money', 'It's easier than medicine' or 'I like inflicting pain'.

Many students are worried that they will sound insincere when they answer this question. The way to avoid this is to try to bring in reasons that are personal to you: for instance, an incident that sparked your interest (perhaps a visit to your own dentist), or an aspect of your work experience that particularly fascinated you. The important thing is to try to express clearly what interested you instead of generalising your answers. Rather than saying 'dentistry combines science, working with people and the chance to have control over your career' – which says little about you – tell the interviewers about the way that your interest progressed. Here is an example of a good answer.

> 'Although it seemed strange to my friends, I used to enjoy going to the dentist when I was young. This was because my dentist explained things very clearly and patiently, and I was interested in what was happening around me. When I was thinking about my career, I arranged to shadow another dentist, and the more time I spent at the surgery, the more I realised that this would really suit me. It also gave me the chance to find out about what being a dentist is really like. The things about dentistry that I particularly enjoy are . . .'

It is **vital** that you do not learn this quote and repeat it at your interview. Ensure that your answer is not only personal to you, but also honest. With luck, the interviewers will pick up on something that you said about work experience and ask you more questions about this. Since 'Why do you want to be a dentist?' is such an obvious question, interviewers often try to find out the information in different ways. Expect questions such as 'When did your interest in dentistry start?', or 'What was it about your work experience that finally convinced you that dentistry was for you?'

Question: Do you know what periodontics is?

Comment: There are a range of other questions closely related to this one, aiming to investigate your understanding of some specific areas of dentistry. It doesn't matter whether you are asked about orthodontics, prosthodontics, endodontics or some other area of dentistry, the point is that it gives you an opportunity to talk about your knowledge of the field. This provides another good reason for carrying out careful research into the field of dentistry before applying and asking questions during work experience. Remember that when you are asked this type of question, the interviewer is not expecting you to have an encyclopaedic knowledge of the area, but is interested in seeing whether you have a solid basic knowledge. It would be worth starting your answer with a basic definition and then, if you have further knowledge or experience of the area, expanding on it. It may also provide another opportunity to discuss a relevant article or current issue that you have seen or to further discuss an experience from a work placement.

Question: I see that you spent two weeks with your dentist. Was there anything that surprised you?

Comment: Variations on this question could include 'Was there anything that particularly interested you?', 'Was there anything you found off-putting?' or simply 'Tell me about your work experience'. What these questions really mean is: 'Are you able to show us that you were interested in what was happening during your work experience?' Returning to the original question, answering either 'Yes' or 'No' without explanation will not gain you many marks. Similarly, saying 'Yes, I was surprised by the number of patients who seemed very scared' says nothing about your awareness of the dentist's approach to his or her patients. However, answering 'Yes, I was surprised by the number of patients who seemed very scared. What struck me, however, was the way in which the dentist dealt with each patient as an individual, sometimes being sympathetic, sometimes explaining things in great detail and sometimes using humour to relax them. For instance . . .' shows that you were interested enough to be aware of more than the most obvious things.

Sentences that start with 'For example . . .' and 'For instance . . .' are particularly important, as they allow you to demonstrate your interest. You should keep a diary of things that you saw during your work experience so that you do not forget and can provide examples. You should then review your diary before interview to refresh your memory.

Question: I see that you try to keep up to date with developments in dentistry. Can you tell me about something that you have read recently?

Comment: If you are interested in making dentistry your career, the selectors will expect you to be interested enough in the subject to want to read about it. Some good sources of information that you may want to make use of are *New Scientist* magazine, the GDC website (www.gdc-uk.org), www.dentistry.co.uk, the BBC news website and broadsheet newspapers. You should get into the habit of checking the news every day to see if there are any dentistry-related stories. Note that the question uses the word 'recently': recent does not mean an article you read two years ago – keep up to date. You could, for instance, say 'There was a recent article in *New Scientist* about the different types of bacteria present in the mouth, only a few of which are responsible for tooth decay. At present, anti-bacterial toothpastes and mouthwashes kill all bacteria, including ones that play a beneficial role. Scientists are now working on anti-bacterials that only target specific, harmful bacteria.'

Question: During your work experience, you had the chance to discuss dentistry with the practitioner. What do you know about the way NHS dentists are paid?

Comment: You must be aware of the nuts and bolts of running a dental practice; in particular, it is worth understanding the difference between NHS and private work and the way that the NHS contract system works. You should also have an idea about what a dentist earns and what proportion of it goes back into running the practice. Similar questions might focus on how much dentists are paid for different types of treatment, or how much NHS patients pay for treatment.

Question: Should dental treatment be free on the NHS?

Comment: Although not specifically about dentistry, this type of question can be useful for an admissions tutor to see how you can think on your feet about wider issues. Obviously this type of question needs you to understand what the issues surrounding the NHS are and to have knowledge of what is going on in the world; but more importantly, it needs you to be able to form and express opinions. There is no way you can memorise an answer to this sort of question, as it is not just about recalling facts. If you are struggling to figure out exactly how to respond to such a question, it is worth taking a moment to gather your thoughts before you respond. It is also worth considering both sides of the argument and expressing your reflection on these, as it shows that you have an appreciation of the range of issues involved.

Question: What qualities should a dentist possess?

Comment: Don't simply list the qualities. The interviewer hasn't asked the question because the interviewer is puzzled about what these qualities are; they have asked it to give you a chance to show that you are aware of them, and that you possess them. The best way to answer this is to use phrases such as: 'During my work experience at the Smith and Smith Dental Practice, I was able to observe/talk to the dentist, and I became aware that . . .', or 'Communication is very important. For instance, when I was shadowing my dentist, there was a patient who . . .'. Always try to relate these general questions to your own experiences.

Question: What is the difference between tooth erosion and tooth decay?

Comment: The interviewer is clearly not asking this question because he or she does not know the answer; it's to find out whether you have learned about common dental problems through your discussions with dentists during work experience. As a prospective dentist, you will be expected to use technical terms more accurately than your friends who do not want to be dentists. A good answer might be: 'I asked this question of my own dentist last time I went to see her. She explained that tooth erosion is the wearing away of the tooth enamel, which can be caused by things such as fizzy drinks (which are acidic) or by grinding your teeth while you are asleep. Decay is caused by the reaction between sugar and the bacteria in plaque.'

Questions about manual dexterity

Question: Dentistry requires a high degree of manual dexterity. Do you possess this?

Comment: The question about manual dexterity is very interesting and often ignored by candidates. Manual dexterity means being able to perform intricate tasks with your hands. Dentists have to work in a confined and sensitive area (the mouth) using precision instruments, in situations where accuracy is vital and where there is little margin for error. If you have trouble picking up a coffee cup without knocking it over or if you always press the wrong keys when you work on a computer, dentistry may not be the best career for you. The interviewers will need to be reassured that you have the manual skills to be able to work on other people's teeth. Good examples of tasks that require a high degree of manual dexterity include sewing, embroidery, model-making, touch-typing and playing a musical instrument.

Manual dexterity is a very important factor that should not be overlooked in the selection process. Students, professionals and admissions tutors to whom I've spoken have all indicated that without this quality a prospective candidate might as well not continue with his or her application. If you are not able to give an example of your own manipulative skills, take up a hobby that involves precision work now, before it is too late. Some admissions tutors like interviewees to bring in examples of their handiwork. A particularly good example of this is a student who brought in a denture that she had made during her work experience. This allowed her not only to demonstrate that she possessed the necessary skills but also to talk about the dental technician's role at a practice.

Case study 3: Sameera Mukadam

Sameera Mukadam completed her A levels at MPW Birmingham and secured a place at Manchester to study dentistry. Her application was particularly strong due to her extensive work experience and voluntary work, her excellent manual dexterity skills and her interview technique.

'I've always loved studying science and knew I wanted to go into a science-related career from early on in my life. I also didn't want a job that involved sitting behind a desk all day, or in an office answering phones; I wanted something stimulating and exciting that involved meeting new people on a daily basis. After an initial work experience placement at a dental surgery I knew dentistry was what I wanted to do – my experiences there really ignited my passion to follow this vocation.

'I then went on to an ongoing work experience placement at a dental surgery for three months during a summer holiday. It was really eye-opening; I came to realise that dentists have to be prepared for all kinds of situations and are more than just someone who will clean your teeth or take away the pain in your mouth.

'During my A levels, I also carried out ongoing voluntary work at a local hospital every Saturday and Monday morning for 18 months. I was involved in sitting and talking to the patients, making drinks for them and also running errands. Most of the people I helped were old and frail and so it was a real joy to be able to help them.

'Once I had applied to study dentistry, I had two mock interviews to help me prepare and understand the types of questions I was likely to be asked. I also carefully researched the details of the courses I had applied to and tried to keep up to date with the latest dental topics so that I could speak about them if asked in interview. I practised answering questions in the mirror and spent a good deal of time talking to myself!

'My first interview was at Leeds and I really enjoyed it. The panel was very friendly and I really felt I had made a good impression. My Manchester interview was the day after and was the toughest interview I've ever been through! During it, one of the panel asked me about how I would make particular one-molar solutions because I had said on my personal statement that I enjoyed practical chemistry. My advice to prospective dentists is to be totally honest when writing your personal statement, because they are likely to catch you out if you exaggerate any particular points.

'In terms of demonstrating my manual dexterity at interview, I took with me a portfolio of pictures I had taken of the henna hand decorating I had carried out. Over a number of years, I had been involved in fund-raisers where I would design patterns for people's hands. I also carried out henna workshops with small children and demonstrated how to do it. My portfolio contained pictures of all of the hands I had decorated and all of the patterns I had designed. I felt that this experience really demonstrated that I had well-developed manual dexterity skills.'

Whatever you do, do not lie about the examples of manual dexterity that you provide. One admissions tutor tells the story of a boy who claimed that he liked icing cakes in his spare time. He brought in photographs of some of the cakes he had iced but it became clear, after very little questioning, that it was his mother who had actually done the work. This did not go down well with the panel, as you can imagine!

Questions to find out what sort of person you are

Question: What do you do to relax?

Comment: Don't say 'Watch TV' or 'Go shopping'. Mention something that involves working or communicating with others, for instance sport or music. Use the question to demonstrate that you possess the qualities required in a dentist. However, don't make your answer so insincere that the interviewers realise that you are trying to impress them. Saying 'I relax most effectively when I go to the local dental surgery to shadow the dentist' will not convince them.

Question: How do you cope with stress?

Comment: Dentistry can be a stressful occupation. Dentists have to deal with difficult people, those who are scared and those who react badly when in a dental surgery. Furthermore, there are few 'standard' situations: everyone's mouth and teeth are different, as are their problems, and things can go wrong. In these circumstances, the dentist cannot panic but must remain calm and rational. In addition, the nature of the profession means that dentists must always be aware of the financial aspects of running a business. The interviewers want to make a judgement as to whether you will be able to cope with the demands of the job.

Having been through this themselves, it is unlikely that they will regard school examinations as being particularly stressful. Hard work, yes, but not as stressful as training to be or practising as a dentist. What they are looking for are answers that demonstrate your calmness and composure when dealing with others. You could relate it to your work experience, or your Saturday job. Dealing with a queue of angry and impatient customers demanding to know why their cheeseburgers are not ready can be difficult. Other areas that can provide evidence of stress management are school expeditions, public speaking or positions of responsibility at school or outside of it.

Question: I see that you enjoy reading. What is the most recent book that you have read?

Comment: An alternative to this question might focus on the cinema or theatre, but the point of it is the same: to get you talking about something that interests you. Although it may sound obvious, if you have written that you enjoy reading on your UCAS application, make sure that you have actually read something recently. Admissions tutors will be able to tell you stories about interviewees who look at them with absolute surprise when they are asked about books, despite it featuring in the personal statement. Answers such as 'Well . . . I haven't had much time recently, but . . . let me see . . . I read *Elle* last month, and . . . oh yes . . . I had to read *Jane Eyre* for my English GCSE' will not help your chances. By all means put down that you like reading, but make sure that you have read an interesting novel in the period leading up to the interview, and be prepared to discuss it.

How to succeed in the interview

You should prepare for an interview as if you are preparing for an examination.

This involves revisiting your work experience diary so that you can recount details of your time with a dentist, revising from the newspaper, website and *New Scientist* articles that you have saved, and consideration of all the things that you have mentioned on your personal statement. The interview panel will have read your statement and the likelihood is that at least one question will pick up on something you mentioned in it. It is therefore vital that you are truthful in your personal statement, as it is very easy to get caught out if you have lied. It is also vital to keep a copy of your personal statement so that you can look over it before your interview; this will enable you to pre-empt some of the points they will raise.

When you are preparing for an interview, try to have a mock interview so that you can get some feedback on your answers. Your school may be able to help you. If not, independent sixth-form colleges usually provide a mock interview service. Friends of your parents may also be able to help. There is a list of some potential interview questions below that you should use to help you prepare. Please note that this is not an exhaustive list, rather a set of questions to get you thinking about your experiences and interview technique. As mentioned previously, do not memorise set answers to questions; this is very easy to spot during an interview and will make you seem insincere. It is much better to have a good idea of roughly what you want to say and then put it across in a natural way. If possible, video your mock interview so that you are aware of the way that you come across in such a situation.

Mock interview questions

- Why do you want to be a dentist?
- What have you done to investigate dentistry?
- Why does dentistry interest you more than medicine?
- Give me an example of how you cope with stress.
- Why did you apply to this dental school?
- Did you come to our open day?
- During your work experience, did anything surprise you?
- During your work experience, did anything shock you?
- Is your own dentist good at communicating with his/her patients?
- Tell me about preventive dentistry.
- What is orthodontics?
- Why do dentists recommend the fluoridation of water supplies?
- What are the arguments against fluoridation of water supplies?
- What are amalgam fillings made of?

- What are white fillings made of?
- There has been a good deal of negative publicity about mercury fillings. Do you think that they are dangerous?
- If you had to organise a campaign to improve dental health, how would you go about it?
- What is gingivitis?
- How are NHS dentists funded? Is it the same for GPs?
- How much does an average dentist earn?
- Have you read any articles about dentistry recently?
- What advances can we expect in dental technology/treatment in the future?
- What have you done to demonstrate your commitment to the community?
- What would you contribute to this dental school?
- What are your best/worst qualities?
- What was the last novel that you read? Did you like it?
- What was the last play/film that you saw? Did you like it?
- What do you do to relax?
- What is your favourite A level subject?
- What grades do you expect to gain in your A levels?
- Do dentists treat children differently from adults?
- What precautions need to be taken with patients who are HIV positive?
- What is an overbite?
- What do you know about forensic dentistry?
- What is the role of the dental nurse/technician?
- How does teamwork apply to the role of a dentist?
- Did the dentists you talked to enjoy their jobs?
- What is the difference between tooth erosion and tooth decay?
- What role does a dentist have in diagnosing other medical problems?
- What do you know about the new/recent NHS reforms for dentistry?
- What do you know about the new government contract for dentists?
- What are the reasons for the increasing use of composite fillings?
- Can you think why dentists might be concerned about the increasing use of composite fillings?

General interview tips

As in any interview, appearance and body language are just as important as the answers you give to the questions you are being asked. The impression that you create can have a big impact. Remember that if the interviewers cannot picture you as a dentist in the future, they are unlikely to offer you a place.

Body language

- Maintain eye contact with the interviewers.
- Direct most of what you are saying to the person who asked you the question, but also occasionally look around at the others on the panel.
- Sit up straight, but adopt a position that you feel comfortable in.
- Don't wave your hands around too much, but don't keep them gripped together to stop them moving either. Fold them across your lap, or rest them on the arms of the chair.

Speech

- Talk slowly and clearly.
- Don't use slang.
- Avoid saying 'Erm . . .', 'You know', 'Sort of' and 'Like'.
- Say 'Hello' at the start of the interview, and thank the interviewer(s) and say 'Goodbye' at the end.

Dress and appearance

- Wear clothes that show you have made an effort for the interview. A suit/jacket and tie (men), or a skirt and blouse (women) are most appropriate and will give the best impression.
- Make sure that you are clean and tidy.
- If appropriate, shave before the interview (but avoid using overpowering aftershave).
- Clean your nails and shoes.
- Wash your hair.
- Avoid (visible) piercings, earrings (men), jeans and trainers.

Structure the interview

It is also possible for you to influence the structure of the interview in the way that you answer the questions you are asked. The selectors will have a set of questions that they may ask, designed to assess your suitability and commitment. If you answer 'Yes' or 'No' to most questions, or reply only in monosyllables, they will fire more and more questions at you. If, however, your answers are interesting and also contain statements that interest them, they are more likely to pick up on these, and you are, effectively, directing the interview. If you are asked questions that you have prepared for, there will be less time for the interviewers to ask you questions that might be more difficult to answer. For instance, at the end of your answer to a question about work experience, you might say: 'and the dentist was able to explain the effect of new technology on dentistry . . .'.

The interviewer may then say: 'I see. Can you tell me about how technology is changing dentistry?' You can then embark on an answer about new types of polymers used in fillings, for instance. At the end of your explanation, you could finish with: 'which will reduce the need for amalgam fillings that contain mercury, which some people believe have an adverse effect on a person's health.' You may then be asked about the possible problems with mercury, and so on.

Of course, this does not always work, but you would be very unlucky not to have at least one of these 'signposts' that you place in front of them followed.

At the end of the interview

You may be given the opportunity to ask a question at the end. Bear in mind that the interviews are carefully timed, and that your attempts to impress the panel with 'clever' questions may do quite the opposite. The golden rule is: only ask a question if you are genuinely interested in the answer (and which, of course, is one you were unable to find during your careful reading of the prospectus).

Questions to avoid

- What is the structure of the first year of the course?
- Will I be able to live in a hall of residence?
- When will I first have contact with patients?

As well as being boring questions, the answers to these will be available in the prospectus. If you need to ask these questions, it will be obvious to your interviewers that you have not done any serious research.

Questions you could ask

- 'I haven't studied biology at A2 level. Do you think I should go through some biology textbooks before the start of the course?' This shows that you are keen, and that you want to make sure that you can cope with the course. It will give them a chance to talk about the extra course they offer for non-biologists.
- 'Do you think I should try to get more work experience before the start of the course?' Again, an indication of your keenness.
- 'Earlier, I couldn't answer the question you asked me on fluoridation of water supplies. What is the answer?' Something that you genuinely might want to know.
- 'How soon will you let me know if I have been successful or not?' Something you really want to know.

Remember: if in doubt, don't ask a question. End by saying 'All of my questions have been answered by the prospectus and the students who showed me around the dental school. Thank you very much for an interesting day.' Smile, shake hands (if appropriate) and say goodbye.

How you are selected

During the interview, the panel will be assessing you in various categories. Whether or not the interview appears to be structured, the interviewers will be following careful guidelines so that they can compare candidates from different interview sessions. Some panels adopt a conversational style, whereas others are more formal.

The scoring system will vary from place to place, but in general, you will be assessed in the following categories:

- reasons for the choice of dental school
- academic ability
- motivation for dentistry
- awareness of dental issues
- personal qualities
- communication skills.

You are likely to be scored in each category, and the dental school will have a minimum mark that you will have to gain if you are to be made an offer. If you are below this score but close to it, you may be put on an official or unofficial waiting list. If you are offered a place, you will receive a letter from the dental school telling you what you need to achieve in your A levels: this is called a conditional offer. Post-A level students who have achieved the necessary grades will be given unconditional offers. If you are unlucky, all you will get is a notification from UCAS saying that you have been rejected. If this happens, it is not necessarily the end of the road in dentistry, as you may be able to reapply as a post-A level applicant. What you must do in this situation is contact the universities that you applied to and ask for feedback about why you were unsuccessful. Some universities will be more helpful than others and give relatively detailed feedback, which will give you points to consider. Others will just send you a standard letter with no details of your particular application.

When UCAS has received replies from all of your choices, it will send you a statement of offers. You will then have about a month to make up your mind about where you want to go. If you only have one offer, you have two choices. One is to accept the choice and go to that university happy in the knowledge that you are going to study the course of your dreams; the other is to reject the choice, if you have decided for what- ever reason that you don't want to go to that university. If you choose to go down this route, you must then apply either the following year or through what is known as UCAS Extra; although it is highly unlikely that places for dentistry will appear on Extra.

If you have more than one offer, you have to accept one as your firm choice, and may accept another as your insurance choice. If the place where you really want to study makes a lower offer than one of your other choices, do not be tempted to choose the lower offer as your insurance since you are obliged to go to the dental school that you have put as your firm choice if you achieve the grades. If you narrowly missed the grades required by your firm offer, you may still be accepted on to the course. You would have to accept this offer so you would not be able to go to your insurance choice. You can only go to this school if your firm choice will not accept you. So, if you had put the dental school you really wanted to study at as your insurance choice, in this instance, you would not be able to accept a place there.

If you are unsuccessful, there remains the option of completing a first degree and then attempting graduate entry or studying dentistry overseas (see page 80).

5 | What do I do on results day?

You will probably have been worrying about results day for a number of weeks by the time it eventually rolls around. Although it can be a very emotional day for some, it is important to be thoroughly prepared to deal with whatever situation may arise on the day.

Your A level results will usually arrive at your school on the third Thursday in August, with the dental schools receiving them a few days earlier. It is vital that you are present in person on the day so that you can collect your results; don't wait for your school to post them, and try to avoid getting them by phone or email as this can sometimes lead to you being given incorrect information. Collecting your results at school will put you in the best position to act as quickly as possible if you haven't managed to secure your place. Prior to results day, check what time your school opens and what time results are available; the sooner you get to your college and pick them up, the sooner you could be on the phone to university admissions teams. In addition to this, you will usually be able to find out whether you have been accepted or rejected from your chosen universities prior to going into your school or college by logging on to UCAS, so have your login details to hand.

If you received a conditional offer and your grades equal or exceed that offer, congratulations! You can relax and wait for your chosen dental school to contact you with details of accommodation and other arrangements.

What to do if you hold no offer

There are a number of students who will approach results day without having received an offer from a dental school. In the past, if you found yourself in this position and secured excellent grades in your A levels, it may have been possible to find a place through Clearing. Unfortunately, it is now virtually impossible for a student to secure a place on a dentistry course in this way, even if they hold outstanding grades. This situation is unlikely to change in coming years. Ultimately, though, Clearing may be of use to secure a place on an alternative course.

If you hold three A/A* grades but were rejected when you applied through UCAS (i.e. you did not get an offer), you need to let the dental schools know that you are out there, and discuss options for how you may secure a place in the future. The best way to do this is by phone or email, as these are the quickest way of contacting the dental schools directly. It is always best to try to establish a good working relationship with admissions tutors and admissions teams at the universities you are interested in, as they will be more likely to give you advice and help you in the future.

In this situation, the main option you have is to reapply through UCAS in the next admissions cycle. Although you will already have the grades for entry in this situation, it is important to understand that there are a number of other elements of your application that you'll need to work on to maximise your chances of securing a place. Things to consider are listed below.

- Your personal statement – revisit it and cast a critical eye over it. This is also an opportunity to add in any work placements or other positive experiences that you have had since your last application.
- Your UKCAT score – you will need to resit your UKCAT for each admissions cycle. This will give you a chance to complete further practice questions and learn from your experience of sitting it first time around. It may also be a good idea to attend one of the UKCAT preparation courses that are available.
- Your work experience – any opportunity to add further work experience to your profile will always be a good step. Whether it is dentistry-related or just general voluntary work, it will have a positive impact.
- Evidence of manual dexterity – if you were called to interview, would you have evidence of your high degree of manual dexterity? If not, the gap between results and applying again is an ideal time to develop an interest that could support this.

Is the Adjustment facility on the UCAS website of any use to me?

In effect, the UCAS Adjustment option is designed to be a 'trading up' system for applicants who pass their exams with better results than expected. However, you can only enter Adjustment if your results have **met and exceeded** the conditions of your conditional firm (CF) choice. A student must have held a conditional firm choice on their application to be eligible and so if you have had no offers, then it is not something you can use.

What to do if you hold an offer but miss the grades

If you have only narrowly missed the required grades, it is important that you contact the dental admissions team as soon as possible. As mentioned previously, you will probably know what their decision is at this point, thanks to the UCAS website. If you have been rejected, it is vital that you keep a level head and do not panic; you must stay calm throughout. If you have not been rejected outright or are unsure of their decision, you must contact the admissions team by telephone – so ensure that in the run-up to results day you have gathered together the contact numbers of the universities you have accepted as your firm and insurance choices.

In some cases, dental schools will allow applicants who hold a conditional offer to slip a grade (particularly if they came across well at the interview stage) rather than offering the place to somebody else. However, be warned – this is a rare occurrence and most of the time dropping a grade will result in outright rejection.

When speaking to the universities, they are likely to give you a simple yes or no answer or tell you that you are still being considered. It is unlikely that crying, begging or pleading your case to the person on the phone will make any difference to the overall decision. If they tell you that you have been rejected, there are some questions you should ask.

- Would they consider your application if you applied next year (i.e. do they accept resit students)?
- What would the likely grade requirements be? (They will almost certainly ask for at least AAA, but it is worth checking anyway.)
- Would they interview you again?

If they have given you a positive response about reapplying, seek to get it confirmed in writing, as this will give you hard evidence of their intention to consider your application again. It is probably easiest for them to confirm this by email, so you will first need to send them an email to enquire. If you are told by the universities you held offers with that they will not consider your application in the next cycle, you should call other dental schools to see if they would consider you. Unfortunately, the number of dental schools that will consider applications from retake students who have not held a conditional firm offer with them is becoming more limited every year (see Chapter 9, Table 2, page 108).

If you have had a positive response from one or more dental schools about reapplying, you would then need to consider retaking your A levels and applying again later in the year (see below). The alternative is to use the Clearing system to obtain a place on a degree course related to medicine or dentistry and then apply to the dental course after you graduate and hope to be offered a place. Remember: as previously mentioned, entry onto dentistry courses through Clearing is no longer an option.

Retaking A levels

The grade requirements for retake candidates are normally higher than for first-timers (currently AAA). You should retake any subject where your first result was below A and you should aim for an A or higher in any subject you do retake.

Take advice from the college that is preparing you for the retake. Most subjects allow you to retake some or all units in January. In some cases, you might be close enough to the grade boundary to risk retaking just one unit; but bear in mind that the more units that you retake, the fewer extra marks you have to achieve in each to reach the magical figure of 480 UMS (uniform mark scale) – the A grade boundary. It is also worth remembering that A2 units are harder than AS units, so you are more likely to be able to gain the extra marks that you need by retaking an AS unit or two than by relying on the A2 units alone.

If you simply need to improve one subject by one or two grades and can retake the exam on the same syllabus in January, then the short retake course (September to January) is the logical option. If, on the other hand, your grades were DDE and you need to retake all three subjects, then you probably need to spend another year on your retakes. You would find it almost impossible to cope with three subjects and achieve an increase of nine or 10 grades within the 16 weeks or so that are available for teaching between September and January.

Numerous state and independent sixth-form colleges provide specialist advice and teaching for students considering A level retakes. Interviews to discuss this are free and carry no obligation to enrol on a course, so it is worth taking the time to talk to staff before you embark on A level retakes.

Reapplying to dental school

Many dental schools do not consider retake candidates (see Chapter 9, Table 2, page 108) so the whole business of applying again needs careful thought and research, hard work and a bit of luck.

When reapplying, the choice of dental schools open to you will be narrower than the first time round. Some do not consider retake students at all; others will only consider you if there are extenuating circumstances that affected your academic performance, while some will only consider you if you previously applied to study with them and were made an offer. It is vital that you check the advice given by each dental school before you think about applying to them, as their position on retake students is always changing.

If you feel that there are extenuating circumstances that have prevented you from reaching your target grades, you must try to get evidence to support this. For example, if you have had a medical condition that has affected your performance, a letter from your doctor will be sufficient. Some examples of acceptable reasons for underachieving are:

- your own illness
- the death or serious illness of a very close relative.

The following are examples of excuses that would not be regarded by admissions tutors as extenuating circumstances.

- 'I had so many exams to revise for that I didn't have time to do everything.'
- 'I have three young brothers and the noise they make stops me from revising.'
- 'I went skiing at Easter, and was unable to revise properly because it was too cold in the evenings for me to work.'
- 'I lost all of my notes a week before the exam and so couldn't revise.'
- 'We moved house a month before the exams, which disrupted my revision schedule.'

These are just guidelines, and the only safe method of finding out whether a dental school will consider your application is to call or write and ask. It is often worth writing a letter so that you have firm details of what has been discussed to refer back to at a later point if necessary. A sample letter is provided on page 74, although a telephone discussion should also take this form. Don't follow it word for word, and do take the time to write to several dental schools before you make your final choice. The format of your letter should be:

- opening paragraph
- your exam results – set out clearly and with no omissions
- any extenuating circumstances – a brief statement
- your retake plan – including the timescale
- a request for help and advice
- closing paragraph.

Make sure that your letter is brief, clear and well presented. You can type it if you wish. If you have had any previous contact with the admissions staff you will be able to write 'Dear Dr Smith' and 'Yours sincerely'. Even if you go to this trouble, the pressure on dental schools in the autumn is such that you may receive no more than a standard reply to the effect that, if you apply, your application will be considered. Apart from the care needed in making the choice of dental school, the rest of the application procedure is as described in the first part of this guide.

52 Boscombe Road
Shufflefield
SH3 2DS
0123 456 7890

Miss A. D. Nash
Admissions Officer
Shufflefield University School of Dentistry
University Road
Shufflefield
SH1 4GH

16 August 2010

Dear Miss Nash

Last year's UCAS No 08–123456–7

I am currently in the process of completing my UCAS application and am particularly interested in applying to Shufflefield to study dentistry. I applied to you last year and received an offer of AAB but missed the grades/was rejected after interview/was rejected without an interview. However I am very impressed by the university and the structure of the course and as such would like to apply again. I have just received my A level results, which were Biology B, Chemistry B, Psychology B. I also have a grade B in AS English Literature.

During my final year of A levels, I had significant health problems that prevented me from achieving the grades I am capable of. I am now embarking on a 16-week course in each of my subjects so that I can improve my grades. Now that I am back to full health, I have no doubt that I can achieve A grades in each subject.

Could you please advise me as to whether you would consider my application, given the circumstances I have outlined above. I am very keen not to waste a slot on my UCAS application (or your time) by applying to you if you will reject me purely because I am retaking.

I am very keen to come to Shufflefield, and would be extremely grateful for any advice that you can give me.

Yours sincerely

Diana Littlewood (Miss)

6 | Other pathways for non-standard applicants

Most students who consider pursuing dentistry at university will be classified as 'standard' applicants; these would be UK residents, studying at least two science subjects at A level and who are applying from school/college or who are retaking immediately after disappointing A level results. However, if you do not fit the profile of a 'standard' applicant but wish to study dentistry, there are other possible options that can be pursued.

Those who have not studied science at A level

If you decide that you would like to study dentistry after starting on a combination of A levels that does not fit the subject requirements for entry to dental school, you can apply for the pre-dental course. The application procedure, the interview and UKCAT requirements are the same as for the five-year course at that particular university. This course is offered at four faculties of dentistry: Bristol, Cardiff, Dundee and Manchester (see Chapter 9, Table 3 for specific details). The course covers elements of chemistry, biology and physics and lasts one academic year. Following successful completion, you automatically move into the first year of the undergraduate dental course.

If your pre-dental application is unsuccessful, the best option is to take science A level courses at a sixth-form college. Both state and independent sixth-form colleges offer one-year A level courses that allow you to cover the necessary A levels from scratch. However, covering A level Biology and Chemistry from scratch in one year and getting the required A grades is a very tough challenge and should only be attempted by the most able students. You should discuss your particular circumstances with the staff at a number of colleges to select the course that will prepare you to achieve the A level subjects you need at the grades you require.

Overseas students

The competition for the few places available to overseas students is fierce and you would be wise to discuss your application informally with the dental school before submitting your UCAS application. Many dental schools give preference to students who do not have adequate provision for training in their own countries. You should contact the dental schools individually for advice.

According to the UCAS entrance statistics, students applying from outside the UK are much less successful than their UK counterparts in getting offers to study dentistry. For entry in 2009, around 65 overseas students (EU and non-EU) gained a place to study at British universities, out of 384 applications. This represents a 17% chance of success compared with a 44% chance for UK students who applied in the same year.

Further breakdown of these figures shows that around 22% of non-UK/EU students gain places, and about 9% of EU students are successful. There are a number of reasons for this and these are discussed below.

Qualifications

Many overseas students are applying with qualifications that are not equivalent to A levels or other UK qualifications, such as the International Baccalaureate (IB), or the Irish Leaving Certificate. These students cannot be considered unless they have done a course that leads to qualifications recognised as being equivalent to A levels. The dental schools' websites will quote entrance requirements in terms of A levels, IB, Scottish Highers, the Irish Leaving Certificate and other equivalent qualifications. If you are studying for other qualifications, you will need to contact the dental schools directly to ask their advice. The UCAS website also has a link to the UK government's education qualifications website, where you can check whether your examinations are suitable.

If not, you will need to think about following a one-year A level programme (studying biology, chemistry and another subject) and applying while studying. Students will also need to demonstrate proficiency in English and in most cases will be asked to have an IELTS (International English Language Testing System) score of at least 6.5.

The application form

Students who are studying outside the UK are often at a disadvantage because they may not have access to advisers at their schools who are familiar with the requirements of a successful application. The two areas that tend to be weakest are the personal statement and the reference. Students who are unfamiliar with UCAS applications often write unsuitable personal statements which concentrate too much on non-essential information (prizes, awards, responsibilities) and not enough on matters relevant to dentistry. It is important to explain why you wish to study dentistry in the UK rather than in your home country. Detailed advice on the personal statement can be found in Chapter 4 of this book. Similarly, your referee needs to be familiar with what the dental schools require in the reference. The UCAS website contains a section on information for referees: you should ensure that your chosen referee is familiar with this.

Work experience

Dental schools almost always require applicants to have gained some relevant work experience, and often to have done some voluntary work as well. Work experience tells the selectors that the candidates are serious about becoming dentists and that they are familiar with what the profession demands. Voluntary work demonstrates that the applicant has the caring nature necessary to work with patients. Gaining work experience can be difficult, but you should make every effort to do so. If it is impossible for you to gain dental work experience, you might try to substitute it with hospital work or by attending relevant lectures. It is important that the reference explains why there is no mention of work experience in the application, and what you did to try to get that experience.

In addition to trying for work experience, there are short courses run in hospitals by dentists giving an insight into the profession. This is particularly useful for those who are not convinced that dentistry is the right profession for them, and also for those who have made up their minds but want greater insight and a good talking point for interview. Visit www.mdexperience.co.uk for further information on these short seminars.

Interviews

Most dental schools require students to attend interviews. This is often difficult to arrange for students who are not based in the UK. It is worth contacting the schools before you apply to see whether they are likely to require you to travel to the UK to be interviewed.

Quotas

While there is no restriction on places for EU students (who will be considered alongside UK applicants), the UK government imposes quotas for non-UK/EU students. For example, Bristol only accepted four non-EU international students for entry in 2009. In general, students from countries that do not have adequate training programmes for dentistry are likely to have an advantage. If you are serious about studying dentistry in the UK, then do not be put off by the statistics. It is worth bearing in mind that while almost all of the UK applicants will be suitably qualified to study dentistry and will be aware of the entrance requirements (academic and other), a high proportion of overseas applicants will be rejected simply because they have not researched the requirements properly. So, careful preparation will give you a good chance of being considered. In 2009, around 52 non-EU overseas applicants were successful, and many go on to have a long and fruitful career, often staying in the UK.

Mature students

Every year, there are a number of entrants to dentistry who are mature students. In 2009, there were around 210 students aged 22 or over who gained entry onto a dentistry course. In general there are three types of mature student:

1. those who have always wanted to study dentistry but who failed to get into dental school when they applied from school in the normal way
2. those who have studied a science-related degree and at some point decided that they wish to study dentistry
3. those who came to the idea later on in life, often having embarked on a totally unrelated degree or career.

The first two types of applicant here will usually have completed a degree in an associated discipline, such as a science or healthcare-related subject and obtained usually a minimum classification of 2.1. This may be because they did not get into dentistry when they applied as an A level student, or simply wanted to pursue a science degree without ever really considering dentistry at the time. If this route is to be considered, an applicant must ensure that they pursue an appropriate first degree such as:

- anatomy
- biomedical sciences
- biochemistry
- human biology
- medical science
- physiology.

This is intended as a guide only and the suitability of any degree course should be checked directly with the university.

This type of applicant would then apply to one of the four-year graduate entry courses following completion of their first degree. This type of course is offered by Aberdeen, King's College, Liverpool, Peninsula and Queen Mary. These courses offer exemption from the first year of the course, so entry is into year two. Students who opt for this path can face an uphill struggle and so would need to have an excellent profile that demonstrates ongoing commitment to dentistry to maximise their chances of entry onto the course.

The second category of mature student is of equal interest to the dental school selectors and interviewers. Applications from people who have achieved success in other, non-science-related careers and who can bring a breadth of experience to the dental school and to the profession are welcomed. The main difficulty facing those who come late to the idea of studying dentistry is that they rarely have scientific backgrounds. There are two possible pathways that can be considered if you are in this position. Firstly, it would be possible to study science A levels and apply for a five-year course. A number of independent sixth-form colleges would be best placed to provide this pathway. Alternatively, it would be possible to apply to one of the six-year dental courses which incorporate a pre-dental year. These courses are offered by Bristol, Cardiff, Dundee and Manchester and are open to those with good A levels (usually BBB or above) that are not in science subjects.

Case study 4: Joanne Lamb

Joanne Lamb is a medical graduate from the University of Sheffield and is currently studying dentistry at Sheffield University as part of her training for maxillofacial and oral surgery.

'I find dentistry far more practical than medicine, with much earlier patient contact and responsibility for patients in terms of treatment planning, booking appointments, lab work and general time-keeping and organisational skills. It is important to realise that dentistry is not as narrow a subject as some people might think; there are a wide range of specialities and also lots of general medicine in the course.

'My advice to prospective dentists would be to use your general life experiences to your advantage on your personal statement. Do not just list your hobbies, talk about what they teach you. Everything can be turned into something positive – a student on an open day the other day asked me whether art A level was relevant as a fourth subject. I told him to definitely mention it as dentistry is very arty – quite a lot of "sculpture" is involved when trying to rebuild teeth. Also, make sure you don't just concentrate on academic achievements in your statement or interview – everyone will have the grades so what makes you different? I would also suggest trying to get some work experience on top of clinical experience – maybe working in a dental tech lab, as this can provide valuable extra background.'

Studying abroad

One option for those who have been unsuccessful with their applications is to study dentistry at one of a number of dental schools abroad. These are five- to six-year courses that are taught in English and are recognised by the UK's General Dental Council. The most well known of these universities are Charles University in the Czech Republic or Comenius University in Bratislava, capital of Slovakia, although there are many others available. Application to these dental schools is not done through UCAS but rather through companies such as M&D Europe (www.readmedicine.com) or Euromed (www.studymedicineabroad.co.uk). Consequently, applicants who are offered a place to study dentistry in Europe are not obliged to accept their place if they later choose to study in the UK. It is advisable for any committed prospective dentist who is applying for a UK dental school to have a back-up option to study dentistry in Europe, in the event that their application in the UK is unsuccessful.

There are two main routes onto these courses. M&D offers a course called M&D Foundation (http://medipathways.com/foundation.html). This is a one-year programme aimed at students with varying academic backgrounds, including those who have not studied sciences. It is taught at a central London location and aims to give students the science groundwork needed to continue their studies at university. Students are required to have achieved at least five GCSEs or equivalent. Successful completion of the M&D Foundation leads directly on to the M&D Pre-Med course. Students need to achieve a score of 65% or above and an IELTS score of at least 6.5 to gain direct entry. The M&D Pre-Med Programme is a one-year course taught in central London and is also available to students who have not completed the M&D Foundation course. It is aimed at students who have been unsuccessful at getting offers for dental schools and seeks to improve the chances of making a successful application to a UK university. It also provides the opportunity to pursue a course at one of the international dental schools. Successful completion of this course may also allow a student to enter the second year, although this varies between universities.

You will usually be required to take an entrance examination for entry onto this type of course. The company that you are applying through will usually provide a revision course to prepare you for the exam; this consists of A level-standard biology and chemistry questions. In addition to this, there may be an interview component, although this again varies from university to university.

Case study 5: Samera Altaf

'I am currently studying dentistry at UMF University in Cluj-Napoca, Romania, and am about to go into my third year. I chose to study dentistry as I have always enjoyed carrying out practical work and using my hands. I also feel that dentistry is a real art and this has always appealed to me. I have also been inspired by observing my brother's career as a dentist and seeing the enjoyment that he always gets out of it. During my A levels, I carried out a number of work experience placements that also gave me a real feel for what it would be like to be a dentist; this just served to further my desire to pursue this course.

'Deciding to study abroad was a daunting prospect initially. Despite having two brothers already established in Romania in their respective courses, I had reservations about how I would acclimatise – not only to university life but also to a whole new country. I was particularly nervous about the language barrier, studying with a different course structure and the cultural and social differences. However, having being there now for two years, I feel the positives of studying abroad far outweigh the negatives; I have met people from all walks of life, learned a new language and found out about a whole new culture. On a personal note, I have acquired more self-assurance and independence since I started studying here. The only real negative is that I am far from family and friends and I find I often miss them.

'So far, the course has been really hard work and there has been a lot to learn and take in. However, I am finding it really enjoyable, particularly my study of subjects such as anatomy and dental morphology. I also enjoy the labs, as they include working with teeth and dental materials, which is very interesting.'

7 | What career pathways exist for dentists?

General dental practitioners (GDPs)

According to the GDC, there were 37,049 dentists registered in the UK at the end of 2009. Of these, some will run their own dental practices, while others will work in larger practices or groups of practices. Some will carry out NHS work, while others may take only private patients. A large number of dental practices will offer both NHS and private treatment. Private patients have a much wider range of treatment available to them, but they or their dental insurance scheme providers pay the full cost – which is determined by the dentist rather than the NHS. As a result, charges for private dental work can fluctuate widely across the country. It is estimated that about one million people have private dental plans.

Regardless of these differences, most dentists follow a similar path after graduation. During their final year at dental school, students need to consider where they wish to begin their career. The path chosen will vary, depending on the individual student's abilities and interests. Many dental schools organise 'going into practice' days for their students, supplementing information available from the BDA.

Students qualifying at a UK dental school must first complete one year of paid vocational training (VT) in an approved training practice. During VT, the newly graduated dentists (known as vocational dental practitioners or VDPs) work under supervision in such approved training practices. VDPs are paid by the NHS, and their trainers are also paid an allowance. Any earnings generated by a VDP go to the trainer. Following vocational training, dentists usually enter an established general practice as an associate or as an assistant.

There is a difference between assistant dentists and associate dentists. Assistant dentists are employed by the practice owner, and are paid a salary; associate dentists are self-employed and responsible for the treatment that they provide, but work in a practice owned by someone else. The associate dentist buys services from the practice owner, such as nursing or technician support, materials and access to patients, paying the practice owner either a percentage of his/her earnings or a fixed monthly fee. In some areas, a number of practices prefer to employ assistant dentists. An assistantship provides an opportunity to work as a full member of the practice team but without the uncertainties of a role as an associate. Associate dentists who work in the NHS are sometimes called 'performers', and assistants are sometimes called 'employed performers'.

At a later point in their career, many dentists decide to acquire their own practice. They can do so by buying an existing practice, starting a brand new practice or becoming a partner in an existing practice. Whichever they opt for, it ultimately means they are self-employed and involved in running a small business. In addition to being dentists they are thus also businesspeople and are responsible not only for the treatment that they provide for their own patients but also for the administration of the practice, and the employment of associate dentists if necessary. This element of a career in dentistry can be an attractive proposition, as it allows a love of dentistry and a flair for business to be developed side by side; however, there can be greater stresses and risks associated with following this path.

A very important aspect of a career in dentistry is the ongoing professional development that takes place; a dentist is responsible for structuring and developing their career at their own pace and in the direction they wish. This means that a dentist is always learning and seeking to develop new skills and knowledge in their profession.

Like medical general practitioners, GDPs have the opportunity to form long-term relationships with their patients and provide them with continuing care. This means that a dentist can develop long-term community links and make a real difference to the area where they are based.

Case study 6 illustrates the experience of one dentist through the VT programme.

Case study 6: Dr Neva Patel

Dr Neva Patel completed her degree at King's College, London: 'When I qualified, I wasn't sure whether I wanted to become a GDP or work in another field, such as orthodontics or paediatric dentistry. I decided to spend a year in the hospital to gain experience in a range of dental fields.

'Working as a house officer was a very comfortable way of being introduced to dentistry – I saw four to five patients a session, and was able to call on experts if and when the need arose. However, I did not particularly enjoy hospital politics, and I also realised that I did not want a career in research, and so I started my compulsory year's training under a dentist in a dental practice.

'I was very lucky with my trainer, who was extremely helpful and supportive. I enjoyed the year at the practice so much that I stayed on to practise there, and have been there ever since. Among my group of friends who qualified as dentists, I was the only one to stay on at the same practice after VT. I started off gradually, seeing perhaps five to 10 patients a day, so that I could spend time on the treatment. At first, I could take up to an hour on a filling, but I soon became quicker and more confident. The big difference between now and when I first started is that I am not worried about what will come in through the door – I feel that I can cope with anything. The job does have stressful times, of course, particularly when dealing with difficult or aggressive patients. However much you are taught about stress management and dealing with anxious patients at dental school, it cannot prepare you for the real thing.

'Some patients can be aggressive because they are scared. I find that the best way to deal with nervous patients is to explain to them exactly what I am doing at all times. Whenever I use a new instrument, I tell the patient what it is for, and what I will do with it. I explain why I am taking X-rays, and the likely lifetime of the treatment that I am performing. Otherwise, they cannot see what is going on, and can become more frightened. The best part of the job, for me, is when my patients are genuinely pleased with the treatment: I find it very gratifying when new patients are referred by existing ones. I also like the flexibility of the job, and the fact that I can control my hours.

'My position is slightly unusual because I am a salaried dentist. This enables me to spend more time with my patients if they need it, and to devote some time to teaching patients about dental health. I don't have to worry about filling my day to maximise my earnings. It means that there is a limit to what I earn, but it also adds to job satisfaction.'

Hospital and community dentists

Hospital dentistry

Hospital dentistry concentrates on more specialist areas such as orthodontics, restorative dentistry for victims of accidents or illness, paediatric dentistry or oral medicine. As a hospital dentist, the career path is similar to that followed by a doctor: junior, speciality and so on, up to consultant level.

Unlike GDPs, hospital dentists receive a salary. Hospital dentistry is thus possibly less risky, as it is salaried full-time employment (see also case study 6). Hospital dentists generally work as part of a team, have access to specialised diagnostic facilities and work with consultants in other specialisations. Another advantage is that, in the hospital service, there is a prescribed and well-defined career structure and training pathway. However, the hours are not as flexible and time will be spent 'on call', resulting in long working sessions.

Salaried primary care dental service

Some newly qualified dentists prefer to follow a more structured path, and choose to become part of the salaried primary care dental service (SPCDS), which provides dental treatment for a wide range of patients with special needs. As with the hospital service, these posts are salaried and there is a career structure, but this option is less structured than working in the hospital setting. It is possible to carry out your VT in the SPCDS.

Having completed VT, experience is gained as a community clinical dental officer (CCDO), with further opportunity to gain postgraduate qualifications through part-time study. Ambitious CCDOs may wish to become senior dental officers (SDOs), with special responsibilities, such as health promotion, epidemiology or treating patients with special needs (see www.nhscareers.nhs.uk/details).

Other careers in dentistry

In addition to the common career paths outlined above, dentists can also find employment in the armed forces and industry. For those with an interest in the academic aspects of dentistry, there are also opportunities for research or teaching in universities. Some dentists will opt for academia and become teachers or lecturers in dental schools and involved in research.

Dental bodies corporate (DBCs)

A relatively new development is the increased possibility of working for a body corporate (i.e. a private dental firm), some of which actively recruit dentists from overseas.

The BDA has an advice sheet on working for corporate bodies, which is available to members. By law, DBCs have to be registered with the General Dental Council. This sector is currently on the increase, due to a general move away from NHS dentistry, a growing consumerism among the general public (e.g. wealthier patients demanding top-notch care) and deregulation of the profession, allowing dentists to advertise, thus making company branding possible. A further reason given by the

BDA is the belief of venture capitalists, among others, that investment in dentistry will yield attractive returns.

Dentistry in the armed forces

According to the BDA, all three defence forces employ dentists to provide a comprehensive service for personnel, both abroad and in the UK. Dentists hold a commissioned rank and there is a very structured career path. If you choose to practise in the armed forces, financial scholarships may be available during your dental studies. It is also possible to carry out vocational training in this sector. For more information on careers in armed forces dentistry, visit the army's website and the Defence Dental Services' website, provided by the Ministry of Defence (MoD):

- www.mod.uk/DefenceInternet/MicroSite/DMS/OurTeams/DefenceDentalServicesdds.htm
- www.army.mod.uk/army-medical-services/radc/5335.aspx

Dentistry in industry

Some large manufacturing and engineering companies (for example oil companies and car manufacturers) offer dental services to their employees. These posts are salaried but the role is equivalent to that of a GDP.

University teaching and research

If you like both teaching and research at university level, there are opportunities in this field. Careers in university dental schools allow you to specialise in a particular aspect of dentistry, which can enable you to pursue research into a particular interest in great depth. University dental teachers will have gained postgraduate qualifications and can progress to become senior lecturers or professors and, if they so wish, get involved with writing teaching materials.

Running a business

Running a dental practice involves all of the skills required in running a business as well as the skills needed to be a dentist. This means that a practice will have to rent or buy a site, employ qualified staff, train them, pay tax and so on. The income of a practice serves to pay the employees, rates and rent. A proportion of the profit is reinvested in the practice for new equipment or new facilities, so that it can continue to offer the best service to the patients. Dentists will be managing a team of people encompassing dental nurses, hygienists, receptionists and others, so good administrative and managerial abilities are needed.

Running a practice can potentially be lucrative, but there are a number of factors that must be carefully considered. These are things such as working long hours, stress and frustrations with the NHS – both of which can be disheartening and unpleasant for a dentist to deal with.

Case study 7: Dr Tom Fraser

Dr Tom Fraser studied at the University of Liverpool. After graduation, he spent a year working at a large NHS practice in Birmingham before joining his father to work in the family practice. He now divides his time between the family practice and a private practice in the Cotswolds that specialises in cosmetic smile enhancements.

'What I find most rewarding about my job is being able to help overcome a patient's anxiety about being treated; this always provides a great degree of satisfaction. I also really enjoy giving patients the confidence to smile! However, as with most professions, there are always challenging aspects of a job that have to be faced on a day-to-day basis. In particular, I find the management of some patients can be very emotionally exhausting. I think it was Lord Winston who said spending a day seeing patients can be draining because you have to give each one a small piece of you; this is certainly true from my experience. On top of the challenges associated with patient care, making sure that administrative tasks are completed can also take up a significant amount of my time and cause some stress.

'In my opinion, one of the most important current issues relating to dentistry is ensuring that all members of the team are adequately trained; it is vitally important that everybody has opportunities to pursue professional development and thereby further their knowledge and skills.

'My tips for aspiring dentists are to work hard to achieve what you want to in your career, but at the same time remember the best policy is to be honest and humble at all times.'

The wider team

Being a dentist in any setting is not just about working on your own carrying out dental treatments; a vital part is working within a team made up of numerous different members. The people who work most closely with dentists are dental nurses, dental hygienists and receptionists/administrative staff. The point of mentioning these team members is to raise awareness of some of the important people that you will need to find, employ and train as a practice partner or owner.

Dental nurses

Perhaps the most important person as far as the dentist is concerned is the dental nurse, who plays a key role in any dental practice. Working alongside the dentist, it is the nurse's job to provide a high standard of care for patients and to be the dentist's assistant. They provide skilled supportive care and are able to perform diagnostic tests such as X-rays.

Dental hygienist

The dental hygienist is also a very important part of the dental team. They are a licensed dental professional with a degree or diploma, specialising in preventive dental care, focusing on techniques in oral hygiene. In most cases, the hygienist is employed by a dental practice. Procedures performed by hygienists include cleaning, scaling, radiography and dental sealing.

Receptionists

The first person you will encounter when you telephone or visit a dental practice is the receptionist. The receptionist is there to manage patients' bookings. In practices where there are multiple practitioners, efficient and effective receptionists and administrative staff are crucial to the viability and long-term profit and health of the practice. In taking care of the appointments process and correspondence at a busy practice, they allow dentists more time to focus on their work.

Women in the profession

It was a little over a century ago that Lilian Murray (later Lindsay) became the first qualified woman dentist, in 1895. At the end of 2009, 40% of dentists registered with the GDC were women, and according to the BDA this figure is expected to rise to over 50% by the year 2020. In recent years, more than 50% of new entrants to dental undergraduate courses in the UK were female; in 2010, just over 55% of all applicants were female.

So in just over a century, women have gone from not being represented in the profession at all to acceptance and potential dominance. Dentistry is a good career choice for a woman and, according to a BDA survey, 93% of women dentists responded that their positive career expectations when entering dental school had been fulfilled. Women leaving dental school expect that, if they wish, they will be able to combine a professional career with caring for a family and/or postgraduate study. The primary reasons for women choosing the profession in the survey appeared to be career flexibility, caring and working with people and the opportunity to combine practical and intellectual work. Anticipated financial rewards did not seem to be a major factor.

Salaries and wages

According to Prospects Planner (www.prospects.ac.uk) a typical starting salary for a dentist in their first year out of medical school as a vocational dental practitioner (VDP) is £29,800 (January 2010 figure). This is expected to increase significantly over the career of a dentist, but the amount it increases will depend on the career path that a dentist chooses. According to the NHS, in 2007–08, the average gross earnings of a self-employed dentist with at least some NHS commitments was £99,208 for a performer-only dentist (one who does not have a contract with a local health body) and £345,651 for a providing-performer dentist (one who has contracts with local health bodies). Before you begin to think about how many Ferraris you could buy when you start earning these amounts, you should be aware that the expenses associated with running a practice (for instance, wages, materials and the practice building) can take on average 52% of this. Therefore, in 2007–08, after deduction of expenses, the average income was £89,062 for a performer-only dentist and £126,807 for a providing performer.

A dentist who opts to work in a salaried post in SPDCS can expect to earn between £37,344 and £79,875 (January 2010). Other salaried posts exist in the armed forces and in corporate practices. In NHS hospitals, salaries at the consultant level range from £74,504 to £176,242 (January 2010).

It is not surprising that, in the private sector, dentists will earn on average around the £120,000 to £140,000 mark after expenses. This can, of course, be far greater, depending on the type of dental practice and the amount of work a dentist is prepared to do. For instance, surgical and cosmetic dentistry are two areas which command the high-end costs of the market.

One factor to consider is that, unlike other careers where earnings rise year after year, dentists often reach a peak in their 30s, and their earnings can fall after this as they become older, slower and less inclined to work long hours.

Case study 8: Dr George Mitchell

Dr George Mitchell qualified as a dental surgeon from Birmingham Dental School in 1976. He has worked at several dental practices and was a part-time Clinical Assistant Dental Surgeon at West Heath Hospital (treating the elderly) for 18 years. His own practice carries out private treatment on adults. NHS treatment is provided for children.

'I'm a GDP, so I carry out a wide range of treatments for my patients, but I have a particular interest in the areas of restorative dentistry, cosmetic dentistry and the dental care of the elderly. There is a long history of dentistry in my family; both my father and grandfather were dentists so my practice is long established.

'There are great opportunities for professional development as a dentist and continually developing knowledge and skills by attending courses and keeping up to date with the latest developments. These are enjoyable elements of the profession. I also really enjoy the interaction with people that the job affords; meeting patients and colleagues and interacting with technicians and dental companies is particularly rewarding.

'There are a great deal of challenges involved in being a dentist; I have to ensure that I provide an excellent level of service for my patients at an affordable price while at the same time keeping costs under control so that I can make a reasonable income. It is also vital to keep up with the ever-changing advances in procedures and equipment.

'Aspiring dentists should realise that when following this vocation it helps if you are hard-working and like helping people; this is not a job that you should do just because of the money. It is also important to understand that running a practice requires a range of skills, as it is really like running a small business.'

Graduate prospects

In a recent study, the Higher Education Policy Institute found that at the end of 2009, 17.2% of male graduates were out of work compared with 11.2% of female graduates. With levels of graduate unemployment set to keep rising and reach record levels over the coming years, it is worth considering whether a dentistry degree will be an asset or a liability in the job market of the future, and what the prospects are for successfully entering employment following the completion of your dental degree and training.

The *Guardian*'s online university guide (www.guardian.co.uk/education/ universityguide) gives data on the number of graduates from each dental school being employed six months after graduation. The general picture here is that the job market for dentists remains buoyant and there is still strong demand; and indeed a very high probability of being employed soon after finishing your education. The percentage of graduates in employment after six months ranges from 97% to 100%, with an average employment rate of 98.6%. Even more reassuring is that there are five dental schools reporting a 100% success rate. This is an amazing statistic, considering the current state of the graduate jobs market.

At this point in time and for the foreseeable future, it seems that a dentistry degree will represent a solid investment and lead to excellent job prospects following graduation. At a time when so many graduates are struggling to find work, this potentially makes studying dentistry an even more attractive proposition than it already was.

8 | What are some of the current issues in dentistry?

As part of your research into dentistry and during your work experience you will probably come across news and other articles about a range of current issues related to the profession. While an awareness of what is going on in the world of dentistry may not be of any use in choosing which dental school to apply to, it is absolutely essential when it comes to your preparation for interview, as you will be expected to have a solid understanding of such issues. The aim of this section, therefore, is to give you an idea of some of these issues and provide a starting point for you to do further research. While you are reading and researching, it is important once again to keep a notebook to hand so that you can jot down anything of interest; your notes will then be the perfect starting point for your revision when you receive notice of your first interview.

The current state of NHS dentistry

What were the 2006 reforms?

The state of NHS dentistry in this country continues to be a hot topic and elicits strong emotions, on the sides of both the professionals and the public. In April 2006, the government carried out sweeping reforms of the system, which were heralded as a new dawn for NHS dentistry and designed to entice more dentists into the service, thereby improving access to dental care. Under the old system, dentists were paid for each treatment they performed (there were around 400 separate charges), whereas the current system gives dentists a guaranteed income for providing a certain number of courses of NHS treatment to any patient requiring care. The reforms also targeted the pricing system and simplified the structure into three bands, as follows.

- **Band 1 – £16.50**
  This charge includes an examination, diagnosis and preventive care. If necessary, this includes X-rays, scale and polish, and planning for further treatment. Urgent and out-of-hours care also costs £16.50.

- **Band 2 – £45.60**
  This charge includes all necessary treatment covered by the £16.50 charge, plus additional treatment such as fillings, root canal treatment or extractions.
- **Band 3 – £198**
  This charge includes all necessary treatment covered by the £16.50 and £45.60 charges, plus more complex procedures such as crowns, dentures or bridges.

Note that in this system, only one dental charge is incurred even if you need to visit more than once to complete a course of dental treatment. If you need more treatment at the same charge level (e.g. an additional filling) within two months of seeing your dentist, this is also free of charge.

Table 8 in Chapter 9 (page 117) shows a list of different costs, taken from the NHS. You will see in the table that all of the procedures listed fit into one of the three bands. A person pays only once – one charge for each course of treatment. For example, for a check-up, X-ray, teeth polish, a simple filling and a crown a patient would pay a total of £198 if they all occurred within a two-month period. This pricing structure was designed to try to bring an end to the so called 'drill and fill' culture and allow dentists to spend more time promoting preventive dentistry.

How were the reforms received?

When the reforms were introduced, many patients welcomed the changes because they felt these would go some way to resolving certain problems associated with accessing NHS dental care, in addition to making the pricing structure clearer. However, the changes did mean that the cost of some basic treatments did increase.

Practising dentists were more sceptical of the reforms; a survey of dentists carried out by the BDA in the wake of the changes revealed that 55% of dentists did not think that they allowed them to see more patients. Before the reforms, according to the BDA, 32% of dentists performed 95% of their work on NHS patients, but this has fallen to 25% of dentists since the reforms. This has led to more than 1,000 dentists walking away from NHS work.

What has been the impact of the reforms?

On the whole, the impact of the reforms has been perceived to be negative, with a number of statistics and comments backing this up. Perhaps the most damning statistic that has come to light following the reforms is that, in the two years following their introduction, one million fewer patients visited an NHS dentist. In addition to this, according to the BDA, 85% of dentists did not feel that the reforms had improved access. A report from the House of Commons Health Committee also stated that the reforms had not solved the 'fundamental problems'. It has also been implied that some dentists are now less inclined to perform more complex treatments such as crowns and bridges because they receive less money for them.

The BDA said the reforms do not give dentists enough time to do preventive work. This has caused strong feelings among dentists, so much so that in some areas up to three-quarters of dentists are threatening to quit the NHS. According to the BDA, the deal states that dentists must carry out 95% of the courses of treatment they currently do to get the same money, which dentists say leaves little time for addressing the causes of poor oral health. One of the key issues has been that some dentists have 'used up' the number of courses they had been allocated prior to the end of the year. This ultimately means that they have to turn away any extra patients as they have been given no further funding to treat them.

One dentist I spoke to commented that the NHS does not allow dentists to practise with full clinical freedom and/or reward them for their work, and that until this is sorted out the NHS will remain unattractive to many dentists. As a result, many focus on private practice because this allows greater clinical freedom and more time with patients. In addition, dentists are able to use the best materials and laboratories because any earnings can be reinvested in the business, so in the end, both patients and dentists are happier.

What is the way forward?

In 2009, an independent review of NHS dental services was published that made recommendations about the way forward for dental care in this country. Professor Jimmy Steele, Professor of Oral Health Services Research at Newcastle University, engaged with dental professionals, NHS staff, patients and patient representative groups to compile this review. The government accepted 'in principle' the recommendations of this review and has been piloting them since autumn 2009. One of the key changes proposed in the review is that the income of dentists will be determined by three factors – patient list size, quality of care and the number of courses of treatment rather than just carrying out a set number of courses. In addition to this, the report suggests that patients need to be provided with better information about available NHS dentists and that the three-band pricing structure should be widened to 10 bands. The full report can be found at: www. dh.gov.uk/en/Healthcare/Primarycare/Dental/DH_094048.

Mouth cancer

What is mouth cancer?

Mouth cancer is historically thought of as a disease affecting mainly older males; however, over recent years, the incidence in women and children has significantly increased. One of the major issues with mouth cancer is that there is poor public awareness of the disease and its symptoms. Mouth cancer can affect any part of the mouth, including the lips, tongue, cheeks and throat and has a number of characteristic symptoms, including ulcers that do not heal within three weeks, red and white patches or unusual lumps or swellings in the mouth. A major problem with being able to diagnose and treat mouth cancer is that many people displaying symptoms will ignore them for a long time, thereby delaying effective treatment.

What role do dentists play in relation to mouth cancer?

Early detection of mouth cancer is one of the keys to successful treatment, which was reinforced by the slogan 'If in doubt, get checked out', used for Mouth Cancer Action Month 2009. This means that regular screening by dentists plays a vital role in the process of diagnosing and treating those with the disease. This further reinforces the idea that dentists are responsible not just for treating teeth; they are in fact involved in every aspect of oral health.

What is the incidence of mouth cancer?

According to the BDA, there are around 5,000 new cases of mouth cancer diagnosed annually and roughly 1,700 deaths each year. The number of new cases is rising faster than almost any other cancer in the UK.

Who is at risk?

There are a number of risk factors associated with mouth cancer. However, chewing tobacco or other similar products is the main risk, with excessive alcohol consumption, poor diet and the human papilloma virus (HPV) also contributing to the risk. Smoking and drinking to excess are a particular problem because alcohol can aid tobacco absorption in the mouth. This can increase the risk up to thirtyfold.

Fluoridation

What is fluoride?

Fluorine is a naturally occurring gas. When fluorine forms a binary compound with another element, this is known as a fluoride. Fluoride ions are found in soil, fresh water and seawater, plants and many foods.

How does fluoride work?

Fluoride is beneficial to both developing and developed teeth, as it decreases the risk of decay. Dental decay is caused by acids produced by the plaque on our teeth, which react with the sugars and other carbohydrates we eat. The acids attack the tooth enamel, which, after repeated attacks, will break down, allowing cavities to form. Fluoride acts by bonding to the tooth enamel, thereby reducing the solubility of the enamel in the acids. Fluoride also inhibits the growth of the bacteria responsible for tooth decay. There is also evidence that it helps repair the very earliest stages of decay by promoting the remineralisation of the tooth enamel. However, fluoride is not a cure-all and the risk of tooth decay can still be increased by other factors such as exposed roots, frequent sugar and carbohydrate consumption, poor oral hygiene and reduced salivary flow.

How was fluoride discovered to be beneficial to dental health?

The earliest work on the benefits of fluoridation was the studies of Frederick MacKay, a dentist in Colorado in the early 1900s. MacKay noted a condition in his patients which was previously not described in the literature: many had a strange brown staining on their teeth. Subsequent research by MacKay and his colleague, D. V. Black, resulted in the discovery that mottled enamel (what we now refer to as dental fluorosis) was due to imperfections in the formation of the tooth enamel. They also noticed that individuals with dental fluorosis had teeth that were particularly resistant to decay. MacKay continued his research and discovered the link between dental fluorosis and the naturally high levels of fluoride in the drinking water in Colorado Springs.

What is fluoridation?

Fluoride occurs naturally in our water supply at varying levels, usually below 1 part per million (ppm). Fluoridation is the process by which the amount of fluoride is adjusted to the optimum level that protects against tooth decay. Where fluoride is added, the natural level is increased to approximately 1ppm.

What are the benefits of fluoridation?

Initially, the main beneficiaries of fluoridated water supplies were thought to be children under the age of five years. In areas where the concentration of fluoride in water supplies is 1ppm, rates of decay and tooth loss in children are greatly reduced. High levels of tooth decay in children are generally associated with areas of social deprivation. This is a pattern repeated throughout the EU and the USA. The best dental health regions in the UK are the West Midlands, an area where over two-thirds of the population receive fluoridated water, and South-East England, which is predominantly an affluent area. The worst areas for dental health are those associated with higher levels of social deprivation, such as North-West England. Children living in socially deprived areas with non-fluoridated water supplies can suffer up to six times more tooth decay than those living in more affluent areas or those receiving fluoridated water supplies. For example, in the poorest communities of North-West England, as many as one in three children of pre-school age have had a general anaesthetic for tooth extraction, and in Glasgow tooth extraction is the most common reason for general anaesthesia for children under the age of 10.

Subsequent research has shown that it is not only children who benefit from fluoridated water supplies but people of all ages, as the effect of fluoride on the surface of fully developed teeth is thought to be even more important. Elderly people, in particular, can benefit from drinking fluoridated water. The decrease in salivary flow with age, combined with reduced manual dexterity, means it is more difficult to keep your teeth clean as you get older. So older people are more prone to root surface decay, which is difficult to treat. As fluoride strengthens adult tooth enamel, it helps reduce the incidence of this type of decay.

Probably the two most important advantages of fluoridated water supplies, as opposed to any other method of combating tooth decay, are that it is cost-effective and, most importantly, that all members of the community are reached, regardless of income, education or access to dental care.

What are the problems with fluoridation?

The only proven side-effect of drinking fluoridated water is dental fluorosis. This is mottling of the teeth caused by a disruption of the enamel formation while the teeth are developing under the gums. It occurs between birth and the age of five years, when the enamel is developing. In mild cases, dental fluorosis is purely a minor cosmetic problem, which is barely visible to either the individual or the observer. It is also thought that mild dental fluorosis may further increase the resistance of the tooth enamel to decay. In moderate to severe cases of dental fluorosis, the colouring of the teeth is very pronounced and irregularities develop on the tooth surface. Whether this is purely a cosmetic problem or whether it adversely affects the function of the teeth is a matter of some debate.

Some research has claimed links between fluorosis and higher instances of bone cancer, osteoarthritis and fractures. However, there have been numerous recent studies by institutions such as the British Medical Research Council concluding that, apart from dental fluorosis, there was no clear evidence that fluoridation of water at the recommended level of one milligram of fluoride to every litre of water caused harm to health.

Other concerns expressed about fluoridation are its effect on the environment, particularly on plants. Fluorides have been used in some pesticides and insecticides and their use is now restricted. Other industrial fluorides are one of the main pollutants in lakes, rivers, streams and the atmosphere.

What are the ethical issues involved in fluoridation?

One of the main ethical issues with fluoridation of water supplies involves infringement of personal liberty, as it effectively medicates everyone without an individual having the choice to refuse. We have no choice of drinking water supply other than through our water company, unless we opt to buy bottled water, the cost of which would be prohibitive for certain sections of the community.

The issue of adding fluoride remains an emotive topic, as demonstrated when the decision was made to fluoridate the water supply of Southampton in 2008. The local health authority decided to introduce fluoridation in an attempt to reduce levels of tooth decay in the city. This plan was carried out in spite of a public consultation that suggested 72% of 10,000 local people were opposed to the plan. As a result, local residents have mounted a legal challenge to the decision, which has the backing of local politicians. Their opposition is based on 'the continuing uncertainties with regard to the long-term health risks associated with fluoridation' and 'the possible adverse environmental effects'.

What is the situation in the UK?

In the UK, around 10% of water supplies are fluoridated. Approximately six million people receive optimally fluoridated water, around 3.5 million of whom live in the West Midlands. Other areas with fluoridated supplies are Yorkshire, Trent, Mersey, Oxford and North-West Thames.

The Water Act (2003) handed the decision of whether to fluoridate water supplies to the Strategic Health Authorities (SHAs) in England and the health boards in Scotland and Wales. The wording states that the decision should be made after 'appropriate public consultation'; a fact that we have seen is not always the case. The Act also means that water suppliers have to comply with the SHA and so have no say as to whether the supply should be fluoridated.

The areas in most need of fluoridated water supplies are those with high tooth decay rates, including Merseyside and other parts of North-West England, Yorkshire, Scotland, Wales and Northern Ireland, plus some socially deprived communities in the South, such as inner London.

Who supports water fluoridation in the UK?

- British Medical Association
- Department of Health
- The BDA
- The British Association for the Study of Community Dentistry (BASCD)
- British Fluoridation Society (BFS)
- World Health Organisation (WHO)
- FDI World Dental Federation

What is the situation in other parts of the world?

According to the British Fluoridation Society, the USA has the most well developed artificial fluoridation programme in the world, with approximately 171 million people receiving optimally fluoridated water. Other countries with fluoridated supplies are Brazil, Colombia, Malaysia, Canada, Australia, Chile and Korea.

What other products have fluoride added?

Several other methods of increasing fluoride intake have been used, including toothpaste, mouthwash, milk and salt. Salt fluoridation was first introduced in Switzerland in 1955 and is widespread in France, Germany, Austria, Belgium, Spain, the Czech Republic, Slovakia and in South America and the Caribbean. This method has the advantage of not requiring a centralised piped water system and gives individuals the control over whether they wish to consume it or not.

However, it is not without its problems: dosage must take into account the other sources of fluoride in the area, ensuring intake is not excessive. The production of fluoridated salt also requires specialist technology. Another consideration is the link between consumption of sodium and hypertension, which would make this method of fluoride intake unsuitable for some individuals.

Fluoridated milk is also available and has been used (with parental permission) for nearly 40 years in primary schools. Around 38,000 children in the UK receive fluoridated milk at school, which has a concentration of 0.5mg of fluoride per carton. However, absorption of fluoride from milk is thought to be slower than from water.

Another problem is monitoring and controlling fluoride administered in this manner, as it is more difficult than with water because of the number of dairies involved. Fluoridated milk's dosage of fluoride also has to be adjusted, depending on whether the water supply is already naturally fluoridated or not. Additionally, a significant number of people do not drink milk for health or other reasons.

Mercury fillings

What are mercury fillings?

Amalgam fillings, which are the silver-coloured type, are the most common type of metal fillings and have been used for around 150 years. They are made of a combination of mercury (50%), silver (35%), tin (15%), copper and other metals. The major benefit of using amalgam is that it economical, hard wearing and long lasting, and as such is ideal for using on molars.

Are there any risks associated with this type of filling?

There has always been a belief that mercury could not escape from the amalgam, but there is some evidence that mercury vapour does escape. Some countries have banned the use of mercury in fillings, among them Sweden and Austria. Critics of mercury in fillings claim that the vapour can cause gum disease, kidney, liver and lung problems, Alzheimer's disease and multiple sclerosis. However, according to the British Dental Health Foundation, dental amalgam containing mercury is not poisonous when combined with the other metals present. It states that 'Research into the safety of dental amalgam has been carried out for over 100 years. So far, no reputable controlled studies have found a connection between amalgam fillings and any medical problem.'

What are the alternatives?

The British Society for Mercury-free Dentistry recommends the removal of amalgam fillings and replacement by composite fillings, but only if precautions are taken to ensure that mercury is not ingested or inhaled. 'White' fillings – made of composite materials or polymers – can be used in place of silver fillings, but they are not as strong and so can often be unsuitable for the back teeth, which are subjected to greater stress than the front teeth. Also being developed is the 'smart filling' – a filling that releases calcium and phosphate ions on contact with acids from the tooth bacteria that cause decay. These ions not only stop the decay, but also help to repair damage.

'Was my treatment necessary?'

Because dentists are paid for the treatment they perform, the more treatment that a patient receives or the more complex the treatment is, the more money the dentist will be able to charge. The question has therefore been raised as to whether dentists provide unnecessary treatment to patients just to make more money. The *Guardian*, in an article entitled 'Do dentists put the bite on patients?', carried out an experiment (albeit a limited one) to test this: a reporter booked examinations at a number of surgeries in London, and the recommendations ranged from one filling and a trip to the hygienist (cost £32.92 then) to two fillings and three replacement crowns (£915 then). Even bearing in mind that dentists have to use their professional judgement as to whether treatment is urgently required or could be delayed, the range of recommended treatment in this particular instance is staggering.

The BDA commented: 'Differences in diagnosis are not unusual. It is a matter of judgement and opinion and much will depend on what the patient wants. If you saw lots of GPs you would probably obtain lots of different diagnoses as well.' According to the BDA: 'A dentist's advice about treatment will depend on a number of factors – whether the patient has been seen before, a dentist's understanding of a particular problem the patient might have, the patient's oral hygiene (which might make certain advanced forms of treatment less feasible), the patient's timescale, and so on.'

There have also been suggestions that some NHS dentists can purposefully stretch out a course of treatment over more than two months to make more money. Under the current contract, if patients have to return to the dentist within two months to finish a course of treatment or have further treatment, the work is covered by one fee. However, if the treatment goes beyond two months, the dentist would be able to charge again. One Welshman carried out a series of attacks on his dental surgery, including leaving a hoax bomb on its front doorstep, because he thought he had been overcharged by the dentist!

In spite of these concerns and potential issues, it is clear that the great majority of dentists are scrupulous about providing only appropriate treatment in an appropriate timeframe to their patients.

The nation's oral health

There has been a steady improvement in oral health in the UK. According to the very comprehensive report by the Office of Population

Censuses and Surveys, 30% of the adult population had lost all of their natural teeth in 1978, but by 1998 this figure had fallen to 13%. In 1998, adults who still had their own teeth had, on average, 15.8 sound and untreated teeth, compared with 13.0 in 1978. The average number of missing teeth fell from 9.0 in 1978 to 7.2 in 1998. The average number of decayed teeth also fell from 1.9 to 1.0. Reasons for the improvement include:

- fluoridation of water
- fluoride in toothpaste
- developments in dental treatment
- provision of preventive and restorative dental treatment
- increased awareness of dental health.

There has been a significant push by organisations such as the British Dental Health Foundation to raise public awareness of the need for good general oral health. This has been achieved by carrying out educational campaigns such as National Smile Month and providing information to the public regarding issues such as mouth cancer and fluoridation. It is important to recognise the shift from talking about good dental health to talking about good oral health; this represents the fact that it is not just the teeth but the health of the whole mouth that is important. Promoting the virtues of good oral health in this way continues to have a significant impact on levels of public awareness.

In 2003, a survey into the health of children's teeth revealed that, although it is continuing to improve, there is a big gap between the best and the worst, and some of this is to do with regional differences (www. statistics.gov.uk/pdfdir/dental1204.pdf).

Professor Liz Kay, Scientific Adviser to the BDA (quoted on the BDA's website), said:

> 'While this report does demonstrate a welcome overall improvement in children's dental health, the gulf between those with the best and worst oral health persists. This report shows that a high percentage of our children still suffer unacceptable levels of tooth decay.'

A report in the March 2004 edition of the British Dental Journal says that children from Asian backgrounds have healthier teeth. According to the report, over 60% of white children have some tooth erosion, compared with under 50% of children from Asian families. In both groups, boys were more likely to be affected than girls. The report highlights the statistical correlation between high levels of sugar in the diet and levels of tooth erosion. Different dietary habits between the two groups, therefore, might be part of the explanation. One of the major contributing factors towards tooth decay and erosion in children is the consumption of fizzy drinks. According to the BDA, the effect of consuming any fizzy drink increases the chance of tooth erosion in 14-year-olds by

220% (and over 90% of 14-year-olds drink fizzy drinks). Children who drink several fizzy drinks a day increase the chance of damage occurring to their teeth by 500%.

At the other end of the scale, the proportion of over-65s keeping their own teeth is continuing to increase, due to better oral care. According to a study carried out by the BDA, less than a third of over-65s currently have their own teeth; however, this is expected to rise to about 50% within 20 years. The concern is that this rise will put greater pressure on dentists to provide ongoing treatment to a greater number of people.

The National Institute for Health and Clinical Excellence (NICE) has published guidelines on the frequency of dental check-ups. The recommended interval between check-ups has been the same (usually six months), regardless of the patient's age and oral health, but Ralph Davies of the BDA, quoted on the BDA's website, said:

> 'The BDA has always held that the frequency of dental check-ups should be based on the individual patient, not a "one size fits all" system. How often you need an examination should be based on what is best for you as a patient and the clinical judgement of your dentist. NICE has also called for more research to be carried out on this subject and the BDA strongly supports this.'

Treatments of the future

Over the past 30 years, the way we have looked after our teeth has vastly improved. We visit the dentist more often, spend more money on dental hygiene products and invest in a wide range of cosmetic dentistry procedures to make our teeth more aesthetically pleasing. As with any other scientific discipline, new treatments and practices are introduced as time goes on that further improve dental and oral care, and consequently dental health and hygiene. Two recent examples are discussed below.

Plasma can replace drilling

Currently, dentists use a drill to clean out bacteria from a cavity before inserting a filling; however, a recent article from the BBC suggests that plasma jets could be used in place of drills in the future when carrying out this procedure. Plasma has many natural forms and can be created when energy is added to a gas, using a laser for example. In this case, the bacteria are destroyed by the plasma, but the surrounding tissue remains unaffected. The study found that the low temperatures killed the microbes while still preserving the tooth, and also that it was possible even when the bacteria were present as resistant 'biofilms' on the dentine. One of the main benefits to the patient of using this technology is that it is a totally contact-free, pain-free method.

Toothpaste-free toothbrush

Currently under development is a solar-powered electric toothbrush that works without toothpaste. The brush contains a solar panel that transmits electrons to the head of the toothbrush, where they react with acid in the mouth; this creates a reaction that can kill bacteria and break down plaque cells. The research team has tested the toothbrush on bacterial cultures and found that it causes 'complete destruction of bacterial cells'. The toothbrush will now be trialled.

It is worthwhile trying to keep up to date with advances such as these by reading relevant newspapers, journals and websites. This will enable you to have a good understanding of where the profession is heading and give you the best possible chance of shining at interview.

9 | Further information

Tables

The tables on the next few pages will give you more information about dental school applications, required grades and typical offers so that you have a clear idea of what each school expects from its applicants.

- **Table 2** presents dental school admissions policies for 2011.
- **Table 3** shows what requirements are needed for students wishing to apply to pre-dental courses in 2011.
- **Table 4** has the requirements for graduate entry to dental school in 2011.
- **Table 5** presents statistics on the number of applicants to dental school in the UK in 2009.
- **Table 6** shows you typical interview styles and lengths for each dental school and how many people will be on the panel.
- **Table 7** shows the number of applicants to dental school over four years, from 2006 to 2010 through UCAS.
- Finally, **Table 8** displays the typical costs for a range of dental procedures for reference.

Table 2 Dental school admissions policies – 2011 entry. Notes to Table 2 can be found on p110

	Standard offer	GCSE requirement	Interview policy	Retakes considered?	Retake offer	Sciences preferred	UKCAT policy
Belfast	AAA + A at AS	Mathematics and either physics or double science if not offered at A level. Best 9 scored, 4 points per A*, 3 points per A.	Approx. 5% (1)	Yes (2)	AAA + A at AS	Two (9)(10) (11)	Required (22)
Birmingham	AAA/AAB + A/B at AS	Chemistry, biology, physics (or double science), mathematics, English language or literature – grade A.	Approx. 35–40%	No	–	Two (12)	Not needed
Bristol	AAB	Minimum of 5 GCSEs grade A*/A including English language, mathematics and two sciences.	Approx. 30%	Yes (3)	AAA	Two (9) (13) (14)	Not needed
Cardiff	AAB	B grade in two sciences, B grade in English language and reasonable spread of grades.	Approx. 20%	Yes (8)	AAA	Two (12)	Required
Dundee	AAA	Whichever of chemistry, physics or mathematics not taken to A level must be held at GCSE grade B. English language grade C.	Approx. 45%	No	–	Two (15) (16)	Required (23)
Glasgow	AAB (with at least BBB at end of AS)	Preference given to applicants with English, mathematics, physics, chemistry and biology (or double science) at GCSE grade A.	Approx. 50%	Yes (4)	AAA	Two (12) (17)	Required
King's	AAA + A at AS	At least B in English literature and mathematics if not offered at AS/A level.	Approx. 30%	Yes (5)	AAA + A at AS	Two (18)	Required
Leeds	AAA	Minimum grade C English and mathematics but higher preferred. Six GCSEs or equivalent including English, mathematics, chemistry and biology or double science.	Approx. 29%	Yes	AAA	Two (12)	Not needed

Liverpool	AAA/AAB	At least seven GCSEs at grade A. Mathematics and English language are required at grade B or above.	Approx. 40%	Yes (6)	AAA	Two (18)(19)(20)	Not needed
Manchester	AAB + B at AS	Five GCSEs at a minimum of grade A (including double science or physics, chemistry and biology) and grade B or above in GCSE English language and mathematics.	Approx. 25%	Yes (7)	AAA	Two (12)	Required
Newcastle	AAB	Five GCSEs at grade A or above.	Approx. 40%	Yes (5)	AAA	Two (12)	Required
Queen Mary	AAB + B at AS	Six subjects at B grades or above including English language, mathematics and science. It is acceptable to resit GCSEs in English language and mathematics to obtain a B grade.	Approx. 30%	Yes (5)	AAAB	Two (18)(21)	Required (24)
Sheffield	AAB	No strict policy, but most applicants apply with all A grades.	Approx. 40%	Yes (8)	AAA	Two (9)(13)	Required

Notes to Table 2

1. Majority of offers made without interview.
2. Only if missed grades by one grade and demonstrated commitment to dentistry at Queen's at first attempt.
3. Considered under exceptional circumstances, from candidates who had firmly accepted a conditional offer from Bristol, narrowly missed achieving the required grades and performed well at interview for the previous admissions cycle.
4. Must have previously applied to study dentistry at Glasgow and gained at least BBC grades at first sitting of A levels.
5. Only if there are serious mitigating circumstances.
6. Only if you had previously held a conditional firm offer with Liverpool and there are mitigating circumstances.
7. Only if you previously held a firm offer for dentistry with them.
8. Priority given to those students who have applied to the course the previous year.
9. Chemistry grade A.
10. One other from biology/human biology, physics or maths.
11. AS Biology at least grade B if not at taken at A level.
12. Chemistry and biology grade A.
13. One other lab-based science (preferably biology).
14. Biology at AS grade A if not taken to A2.
15. Biology.
16. Two from chemistry, physics or maths.
17. AS English is strongly recommended.
18. At least biology or chemistry to A level, the other to AS level.
19. Acceptable sciences are: physics, chemistry, biology, maths and psychology.
20. If not offered at A level, either chemistry or biology must be offered at AS level grade B.
21. One other science at A level if not offering both biology and chemistry.
22. Additional point given to GCSE grade score for every section of UKCAT where the result is above average and a point taken away if the result is below average.
23. Secondary to academic performance and interview performance.
24. Applicants are ranked according to their UKCAT score.
25. Cut-off score determined based on number of applicants and their scores.

Table 3 Pre-dental course entry requirements 2011

University	Standard offer	GCSE requirements	A level subject requirements
Bristol	AAB	Minimum of five A/A* grades at GCSE to include English language, mathematics and two science subjects.	Three non-science subjects, or one science and two non-science subjects (excluding chemistry, physics and general studies).
Cardiff	AAB	English or Welsh language at grade B, plus two chemistry, physics or biology. double science acceptable at BB grades.	AAB grades required with no more than one science (excluding general studies).
Dundee	AAA	English language and preferably biology.	No more than one science A level.
Manchester	ABB	English language – grade B or above.	i) Three arts subjects at A2 level or ii) Two arts subjects and one science subject (not including chemistry) or iii) One arts subject and two science subjects (not including chemistry). General studies is excluded

Table 4 Graduate entry requirements 2011

	Pre-degree requirements	Degree requirements	Interview	UKCAT?
Aberdeen	None	An upper second class honours in a medical science degree or an MBChB is also accepted.	Yes	Yes
King's	None	At least an upper second class honours degree in a biomedically related or health professional subject or a lower second class honours degree in a biomedically related or health professional subject with a postgraduate degree (with at least a merit).	Yes	Yes
Liverpool	Three A levels at C or above, two of which must be sciences (geography and sociology are not acceptable). GCSE maths and English language must be offered by all candidates at grade C or above.	Biomedical sciences degree (minimum upper second for classified degrees) or an MBChB from an approved institution.	Yes	No
Peninsula	None	A good honours degree (normally minimum of an upper second class honours degree) in a biomedically related or healthcare professional subject or relevant experience of working as a healthcare professional.	Yes	No, but graduate medical school admissions test (GAMSAT) required if not holding a relevant degree.
Queen Mary	None	Graduates will need a science or health-related degree at an upper second class honours degree or above.	Yes	Yes

Table 5 Dental school statistics – an example of the number of applicants to dental schools in 2009

	Applicationss	Interviews	Offers	Accepted	Clearing	Graduates	Overseas	Resits
Belfast	179	11	70	46	1	4	0	8
Birmingham	962	350	140	75	0	3 to 5	0	0
Bristol	819	236	202	80	2	11*	4	Not available
Cardiff	936	171	152	77	3 (overseas)	0	4	4
Dundee	335	150	144	67	0	3	4	0
Glasgow	463	260	148	92	0	10	5	Not available
King's	967*	270*	185*	128*	0*	15*	10*	0*
Leeds	1352	386	202	81	0	2	3	5
Liverpool	883	358	221	66	0	3	6	6
Manchester	876*	230*	153*	76*	0*	6*	4*	4*
Newcastle	630	260	219	84	0	12	4	3
Queen Mary	1147	275	194	55	0	20	5	Not available
Sheffield	1095	421	176	76	0	2	5	8

* = no new data available

Table 6 Typical interviews – 2011 entry

	Length	Number on panel	Composition of panel	Other information
Belfast	30 mins	4	Multiple mini interviews conducted by a range of staff.	None
Birmingham	15 mins	2/3	Admissions tutor and dental school staff.	None
Bristol	20 mins	2	University and hospital staff who have teaching contact with undergraduates. At least one member of the panel is clinically qualified.	You will be asked to bring along evidence of activities which require manual dexterity. At the end of the admissions tutor's talk, applicants are asked to take a 10-minute written exercise on a topical, dentally related subject (examples are not available to applicants prior to interview). This is used to determine spontaneity, written content, clear thought processes plus use of grammar and punctuation. It is available to interviewers and is scored by the dental admissions tutor following interview.
Cardiff	15–20 mins	2	Academic staff members of the same ranking.	None
Dundee	20–25 mins	2	Members of the dental school teaching staff.	None
Glasgow	15–20 mins	2	Two members of the admissions committee (qualified dentists) or one member of committee and one member of staff involved with dentistry.	None

Table 6 Continued

	Length	Number on panel	Composition of panel	Other information
King's	20 mins	2	Two interviewers who are usually both members of clinical staff or lecturers from the Dental Institute.	None
Leeds	20 mins	3	Each interview panel will normally comprise three members: a dentally qualified staff member, another dental academic and a senior dental student (normally from the fourth or fifth year of the programme).	None
Liverpool	15–20 mins	2	Panels of interviewers are drawn from members of staff in the School of Dentistry, senior dental students, local dentists and local school teachers.	None
Manchester	15 mins	2/3	Practising clinicians. A third member may be present to act as chairman.	None
Newcastle	20–25 mins	2	Members of academic staff on the panel, at least one of whom will be a clinician.	None
Queen Mary	30–40 mins	3	Two members of senior academic or clinical staff plus a third or fourth-year student.	You will watch a DVD and be asked for your observations on its content. There are no 'right' or 'wrong' answers.
Sheffield	15 mins	3	The panel comprises a member of academic staff who is clinically qualified, a non-clinical member of academic staff and a fourth or fifth-year current dental student.	None

Table 7 Applicants through UCAS to dentistry by the October deadline – 2006–10

Year	Total applicants	Male – UK	Female – UK	Male – EU	Female – EU	Male – Non-EU	Female – Non-EU
2006	2,911	1,154	1,310	74	121	111	141
2007	3,114	1,224	1,463	83	114	106	124
2008	2,995	1,209	1,388	70	112	80	136
2009	3,304	1,287	1,558	70	120	93	176
2010	3,720	1,438	1,727	95	178	117	165
Change 2009–2010 (%)	13	12	11	36	48	26	–6

Table 8 Dental procedure costs

Dental work required	NHS prices
Apicoectomy	£198.00
Braces	£198.00
Dental crown	£198.00
Dental examination	£16.50
Dentures	£198.00
First consultation	£16.50
Large tooth filling	£121.80
Root canal	£198.00
Sedated tooth removal	£45.60
Small tooth filling	£45.60
Scale and polish	£16.50
X-ray	£16.50

Source: Reprinted with kind permission from www.whatprice.co.uk/dentist/nhs-prices.html

Postgraduate deaneries in the UK

Defence

Surgeon Captain Adrian Jordan
Defence Postgraduate Dental Dean

DPDD
DPMD DMS Whittington
Whittington Bks
Lichfield WS14 9PY
Website: www.mod.uk/DefenceInternet/AboutDefence/WhatWeDo/
HealthandSafety/DDS

Eastern

Alex Baxter
Director of Postgraduate Dental Education

East of England Multi-Professional Deanery
CPC1
Capital Park
Fulbourn
Cambridge CB21 5XE
Website: www.eoedeanery.nhs.uk/
Tel: 01223 743300
Fax: 01223 743301

London

Elizabeth Jones
Dean of Postgraduate Dentistry

Dental Department
LPMDE
Stewart House
32 Russell Square
London WC1B 5DN
Website: www.londondeanery.ac.uk
Tel: 020 7866 3100

Mersey

Brian Grieveson
Dean of Postgraduate Dental Education & Training

Postgraduate Dental Education & Training
1st Floor
Regatta Place
Brunswick Business Park
Summers Road
Liverpool L3 4BL
Website: www.merseydeanery.nhs.uk
Tel: 0151 285 4700/4701
Fax: 0151 285 4703

North

Malcolm Smith
Acting Postgraduate Dental Dean

Northern Deanery
Waterfront 4
Goldcrest Way
Newburn Riverside
Newcastle-upon-Tyne NE15 8NY
Website: www.northerndeanery.org
Tel: 0191 210 6400 (main switchboard)
Fax: 0191 210 6401 (reception)

North West

Nicholas Taylor
Director of Postgraduate Dental Education

University of Manchester
Department of Postgraduate Medicine & Dentistry

Dental Section
4th Floor
Barlow House
Minshull Street
Manchester M1 3DZ
Website: www.nwpgmd.nhs.uk
Tel: 0845 050 0194 (main North Western Deanery switchboard)

Northern Ireland

David Hussey
Postgraduate Dental Dean

NIMDTA
Beechill House
42 Beechill Road
Belfast BT8 7RL
Website: www.nimdta.gov.uk
Tel: 028 9040 0000

Oxford

Helen Falcon
Postgraduate Dental Dean

Oxford University
Oxford Postgraduate Medical & Dental Education
The Triangle
Roosevelt Drive
Headington
Oxford OX3 7XP
Website: www.oxforddeanery.nhs.uk
Tel: 01865 740601
Fax: 01865 740636

Scotland

Jim Rennie
Postgraduate Dental Dean

NHS Education for Scotland
Thistle House
91 Haymarket Terrace
Edinburgh EH12 5HE
Website: www.nes.scot.nhs.uk
Tel: 0131 313 8000
Fax: 0131 313 8001

South

Stephen Lambert-Humble
Dean of Postgraduate Dentistry

The Dental Department
KSS Postgraduate Deanery
7 Bermondsey Street
London SE1 2DD
Website: http://dental.kssdeanery.org
Tel: 020 7415 3400

South West

Alasdair Miller
Regional Postgraduate Dental Dean

University of Bristol
Regional Dental Postgraduate Department
The Chapter House
Bristol Dental Hospital
Lower Maudlin Street
Bristol BS1 2LY
Website: www.bristol.ac.uk/dentalpg
Tel: 0117 342 4524
Fax: 0117 342 4526

South Yorkshire/East Midlands

Chris Franklin
Postgraduate Dental Dean

Regional Postgraduate Dental Education Office
Don Valley House
Savile Street East
Sheffield S4 7UQ
Website: www.pgde-trent.co.uk
Tel: 0114 226 4454
Fax: 0114 226 4468

Wales

Jon Cowpe
Postgraduate Dental Dean

Cardiff University
Dental Postgraduate Department
Room 130 Dental School

Heath Park
Cardiff CF14 4XY
Website: www.cardiff.ac.uk/pgmde/dental
Tel: 029 2068 7497
Fax: 029 2068 7455

Wessex

Vicky Osgood
Postgraduate Dean

Southern House
Otterbourne
Winchester SO21 2RU
Website: www.wessexdeanery.nhs.uk
Tel: 01962 718400
Fax: 01962 718401

West Midlands

Karen Elley
Postgraduate Dental Dean

NHS West Midlands
St Chad's Court
213 Hagley Rd
Edgbaston
Birmingham B16 9RG
Website: www.westmidlandsdeanery.nhs.uk/Dentistry.aspx
Tel: 0121 695 2555
Fax: 0121 695 2578

Yorkshire

Paul Cook
Regional Postgraduate Dental Dean

The Department for NHS Postgraduate Medical and Dental Education
Willow Terrace Road
University of Leeds
Leeds LS2 9JT
Website: www.yorksandhumberdeanery.nhs.uk/dentistry
Tel: 0113 343 1557

Further reading

There is a wealth of information available both on the internet and beyond. Try to keep up to date with some of the key developments, as this will give you an excellent overview of what is happening in the world of dentistry.

An essential starting point is the BDA's website (www.bda.org). This carries careers information for prospective dentists as well as press releases and discussion of topical issues. The BDA's website for dental patients (www.bdasmile.org) is also useful.

The BDA has its own museum, the BDA Dental Museum, which gives an interesting historical overview of dentistry; details can be found at www.bda.org/museum.

Some other useful websites are www.dentistry.co.uk, www.dental-health.org.uk, www.gdc-uk.org and www.3dmouth.org. These all have a wealth of factual information and details of current issues in dentistry, and as such are worth a regular look, while www.admissionsforum.net is a chatroom for potential medical and dental applicants and has a number of interesting discussions; however, double check any information you receive from here as it may not always be reliable.

The BDA publishes a journal for dentists, the *British Dental Journal* (www.bdj.co.uk). The journal is aimed at practising dentists, and can be very technical; although it does give very nice, short summaries of some of the most relevant hot topics. The International Society for Fluoride Research publishes its own journal called *Fluoride*. Some articles from the journal are available on the society's website (www.fluorideresearch.org).

To keep up to date with dentistry and dental issues in the UK, the *Independent*, the *Guardian*, the *Daily Telegraph* and *The Times* all carry regular health reporting, and have health sections once a week. Another source of dental news is the website www.topix.net/business/dental, which covers topical dentistry stories from the UK and worldwide.

For summaries of course information and academic requirements, a useful reference point is *HEAP 2012: University Degree Course Offers*, written by Brian Heap and published by Trotman (www.trotman.co.uk).

If you are thinking of studying dentistry overseas, M&D Europe is a good source of information. It aims to help you get a place on a course taught in English – and, once you have qualified, to help you get placements at hospitals in the UK. Its website, www.readmedicine.com, gives details of dental schools in the Czech Republic, Spain and Slovakia.

Contact details

Organisations

British Dental Association
64 Wimpole Street
London W1G 8YS
Website: www.bda.org
Tel: 020 7935 0875
Fax: 020 7487 5232

British Fluoridation Society
Ashton Leigh & Wigan PCT
Bryan House
Standishgate
Wigan WN1 1AH
Website: www.bfsweb.org
Tel: 01942 483099

British Medical Association
BMA House
Tavistock Square
London WC1H 9JP
Website: www.bma.org.uk
Tel: 020 7387 4499

General Dental Council
37 Wimpole Street
London W1G 8DQ
Website: www.gdc-uk.org
Tel: 020 7887 3800

Dental schools

University of Aberdeen
Admissions Tutor: Dr Christine Kay
Admissions Secretary: Ms Emma Dunlop
School of Medicine and Dentistry
3rd Floor
Polwarth Building
Foresterhill
Aberdeen AB25 2ZD
Website: www.abdn.ac.uk/medicine-dentistry/medical-dental/programmes/
dentistry
Tel: 01224 559087

University of Birmingham
Admissions Tutor: Mr Donald Spence
Admissions Secretary: Ms Frances Deen

The School Of Dentistry
University Of Birmingham
St Chad's Queensway
Birmingham B4 6NN
Website: www.dentistry.bham.ac.uk/home
Tel: 0121 237 2761
Fax: 0121 625 8815

University of Bristol
Admissions Tutor: Dr John Moran
Admission Secretary: Mrs Geraldine Vines
School of Oral and Dental Sciences
Lower Maudlin Street
Bristol BS1 2LY
Website: www.bristol.ac.uk/dental
Tel: 0117 928 9000

Cardiff University
Admissions Tutor: Dr Robert McAndrew
Admissions Officer: Mrs Victoria Ocock
Cardiff University
Heath Park
Cardiff CF14 4XY
Website: www.cardiff.ac.uk/dentl/index.html
Tel: 029 2074 5867/2468

University of Dundee
Admissions Tutor: Dr John Drummond
Admissions Secretary: Mr Gordon Black
Dundee Dental School
University of Dundee
Park Place
Dundee DD1 4HN
Website: www.dundee.ac.uk/dentalschool
Tel: 01382 344697

University of Glasgow
Admissions Tutor: Dr Christine Goodall
Admissions Secretary: Ms Jennifer Leitch
Glasgow Dental Hospital & School
378 Sauchiehall Street
Glasgow G2 3JZ
Website: www.gla.ac.uk/departments/dentalschool
Tel: 0141 211 9600
Fax: 0141 331 2798

King's College London
Admissions Tutor: Dr Lyndon Cabot
Dental Institute

King's College London
Hodgkin Building
Guy's Campus
London Bridge
London SE1 1UL
Website: www.kcl.ac.uk/schools/dentistry
Tel: 020 7848 6512

University of Leeds
Admissions Tutor: Dr Simon Wood
School of Dentistry
Leeds Dental Institute
Clarendon Way
Leeds LS2 9LU
Website: www.leeds.ac.uk/dental/index.html
Tel: 0113 343 6199

University of Liverpool
Admissions Tutor: Miss Eileen Theil
Admissions Secretary: Miss Abigail Watkins
The School of Dental Sciences
Liverpool University Dental Hospital
Pembroke Place
Liverpool L3 5PS
Website: www.liv.ac.uk/dental/index.htm
Tel: 0151 706 5298

University of Manchester
Admissions Tutor: Dr Anthony Mellor
Admissions Secretary: Ms Teresa Smith
School of Dentistry
The University of Manchester
Higher Cambridge Street
Manchester M15 6FH
Website: www.dentistry.manchester.ac.uk
Tel: 0161 306 0220

Newcastle University
Admissions Tutor: Dr David Brown
Admissions Co-ordinator: Ms Michelle Smith (Mon–Wed only; please
speak to Dr Brown at other times)
School of Dental Sciences
Framlington Place
Newcastle University
Newcastle-upon-Tyne NE2 4BW
Website: www.ncl.ac.uk/dental
Tel: 0191 222 8347

Peninsula College of Medicine and Dentistry
Senior Admissions Co-ordinator: Mrs Susan Davey
Peninsula College of Medicine & Dentistry
John Bull Building
Plymouth PL6 8BU
Website: www.pcmd.ac.uk/dentistry.php
Tel: 01752 437444
Fax: 01752 517842

Queen Mary (Barts and the London School of Medicine and Dentistry)
Admissions Tutor: Dr Christopher Mercer
Admissions Secretary: Mr Jeremy Luz
Barts and The London School of Medicine & Dentistry
Queen Mary, University of London
Garrod Building
Turner Street
London E1 2AD
Website: www.dentistry.qmul.ac.uk
Tel: 020 7882 8478/2240

Queen's University Belfast
Admissions Administrator: Mr Liam Barton
Centre for Dental Education
Grosvenor Road
Royal Victoria Hospital
Belfast BT12 6BP
Website: www.qub.ac.uk/schools/mdbs/dentistry
Tel: 028 9097 3838
Fax: 028 9043 8861

University of Sheffield
Admissions Tutor: Mr Duncan Wood
Admissions Secretary: Mrs Amanda Okrasa
The School of Clinical Dentistry
University of Sheffield
19 Claremont Crescent
Sheffield S10 2TA
Website: www.sheffield.ac.uk/dentalschool
Tel: 0114 271 7801/7808
Fax: 0114 279 7050l1

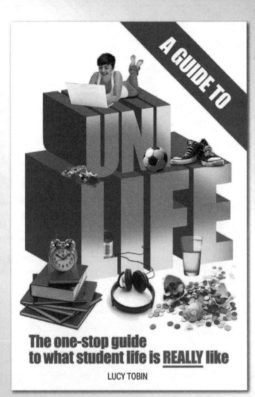
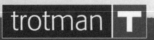

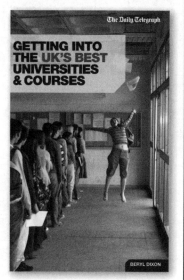
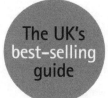
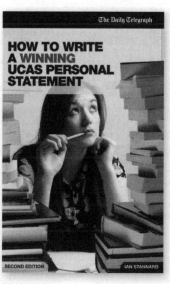

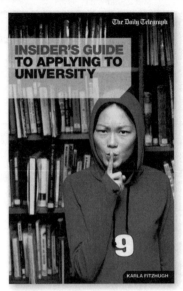
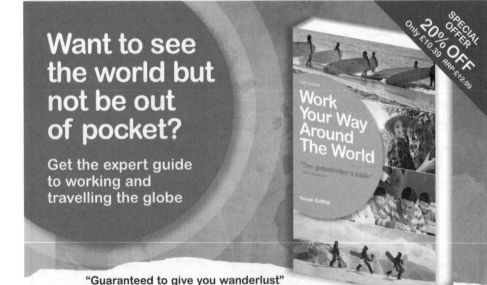

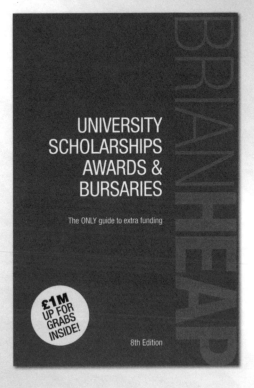
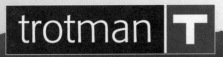